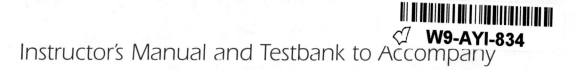
Instructor's Manual and Testbank to Accompany

CLINICAL DRUG
THERAPY

RATIONALES FOR NURSING PRACTICE

therapy, and whether the group is relatively dynamic or stable over time (e.g., new cardio-vascular drugs are frequently introduced).

5. Use the review and application exercises at the end of each chapter of the text.
   a. Select one or more exercises to discuss in class.
   b. Have students individually write answers to one or more, in class or as a homework assignment.
   c. Assign students to small groups (4–6 students each) and have the groups discuss selected exercises and report to the total group.

6. Make an overhead transparency of selected work-sheets and have the class complete the work-sheets as an in-class exercise to stimulate and reinforce learning.

7. Assign worksheets from the *Study Guide* as home-work. Discuss answers in class.

8. Discuss critical thinking case study exercises (in most chapters of the *Study Guide*) as a class or in small groups. For the more complex exercises, an out-of-class written assignment may be more appropriate.

9. Have students complete a medication history on a client, friend, or family member and identify information important in nursing care.

10. Provide portions of nursing process information and have students use the information in plan-ning nursing care.
   a. State a client's medical diagnosis and selected signs and symptoms, then ask students to identify laboratory or other diagnostic test data needed to evaluate the client's response to drug therapy.
   b. Provide a completed medication history, dis-cuss other information, then have students state nursing diagnoses and goals.
   c. State one or more nursing diagnoses and have students state or write the interven-tions needed.
   d. Give students a list of diseases or signs and symptoms of a client and ask them to predict the type of drug or an individual drug that is likely to be prescribed.
   e. Give students a list of a client's drugs and ask them to predict the disease processes or signs and symptoms the client is probably experiencing.
   f. Give students a copy of an instruction sheet from a hospital or community pharmacy. Have students individualize the instructions for an elderly client, a child, someone with renal impairment, etc.

11. Have students "adopt-a-drug" related to course content and write a short paper in which the drug, its "family," clinical indications for use, adverse effects, client teaching implications, and other pertinent information are included. This is an opportunity to be creative and imaginative! Students often choose a drug with which they have had some personal experience, or drug names may be randomly drawn from a container. Prototypes or commonly used drugs are especial-ly helpful.

12. Invite an occasional guest speaker if feasible. Pos-sibilities include a pharmacist from a hospital or community drug store; a nutrition teacher or dietitian; a nurse colleague with expertise in drug therapy with children, elderly, mentally ill, or other special populations; a nurse colleague with expertise in cardiovascular drugs, emergency or critical care drugs, or drug abuse and dependen-cy; a diabetic and family member; a member of a local senior citizen's group; or a member of a local support group for people with various dis-ease processes or drug therapy regimens.

9. Discuss nursing process implications of administering or supervising drug therapy in the home setting.

10. Describe selected legal, ethical, and economic aspects of drug therapy.

11. Evaluate over-the-counter drugs for personal use or instruction of clients.

TOPICAL OUTLINE OF UNITS

I.   Introduction to drug therapy

II.   Drugs affecting the central nervous system

III. Drugs affecting the autonomic nervous system

IV.   Drugs affecting the endocrine system

V.   Nutrients, fluids, and electrolytes

VI.   Drugs used to treat infections

VII. Drugs affecting the immune system

VIII. Drugs affecting the respiratory system

IX.   Drugs affecting the cardiovascular system

X.   Drugs affecting the digestive system

XI.   Drugs used in special conditions

TEACHING METHODS

Audiovisuals   Case study analysis

Lecture/discussion   Nursing process exercises

Recommended readings   Required readings

Small group assignments   *Study Guide* assignments

Worksheets   Written assignments

GRADING POLICIES

ATTENDANCE POLICIES

GENERAL OBSERVATIONS

1. Pharmacology is a basic science on a par with physiology, microbiology, chemistry, and so forth. Thus, similar study skills and time commitments are needed for learning and applying drug knowledge.

2. Students often say they feel overwhelmed by the number of drugs and amount of information they're expected to assimilate and apply to clinical practice. This seems to be a universal and growing problem as the number of commonly used drugs continues to expand. Despite widespread agreement among nursing faculty about emphasizing prototypes, several important drug groups do not have clear-cut prototypes or the prototypical drug is no longer commonly used. Although emphasizing prototypes is usually desirable, limiting

instruction to prototypes does not adequately reflect the diversity and complexity of drug therapy in the clinical setting. Thus, each faculty group or individual instructor must decide which drugs to include or emphasize.

GENERAL TEACHING STRATEGIES

1. Provide students with a vocabulary list (terms and concepts) for each unit of instruction. Terms and concepts may be studied independently, used as a basis for classroom questioning and discussion, or used for written assignments when considered complex or vital to understanding course content.

2. Provide students with a list of individual drugs for each unit of instruction. For students, the drug list can limit the number of drugs to be studied (e.g., a few from each chapter), delineate the drugs they are expected to know, and focus study efforts on important drugs. For instructors, the drug list can guide lectures, discussion topics, test items, and clinical teaching.

   a. List drugs by the generic name and one or more trade names. The generic name is especially important. However, students need to become accustomed to both names because drugs may be ordered by either one. Pharmacies and health care agencies vary in the trade names of drugs they dispense. Thus, the instructor may use trade names that are commonly used in students' clinical practice settings.

   b. The number of trade names in the text is necessarily limited because of space and other considerations. The instructor may suggest that students write in trade names of drugs they often encounter in clinical practice.

3. Provide students with learning objectives for each group of drugs or each class period. These can be written by the instructor or assembled from chapter objectives in this manual, with objectives added or deleted as desired. Students can use the objectives to further their understanding of the instructor's expectations and to guide their study efforts. Instructors can use the objectives as an outline for a lecture, as topics for class or small group discussion, or as topics for written homework assignments to be turned in and graded.

4. Focus activities to get students' attention at the beginning of class.

   a. Introduce the "topic of the day."

   b. Show transparencies of drug-related cartoons or comic strips.

   c. Start class with drug-related current events or "Drugs in the News" (often in newspapers). Ask students to contribute items.

   d. Describe the historical development of a drug or drug group. Useful information may include date approved by the FDA, the impact on drug

Overview and General Teaching Strategies

OVERVIEW

One purpose of this manual is to facilitate the use of *Clinical Drug Therapy: Rationales for Nursing Practice* and its accompanying *Study Guide* in teaching nursing pharmacology. A second purpose is to assist the instructor in evaluating students' knowledge of drug information and their ability to apply that information in client-care situations.

To fulfill the first purpose, a variety of materials are presented so the instructor can custom-design learning activities for a wide range of students. These materials include:

1. A sample syllabus for a separate pharmacology course. This syllabus has been used by the author, with relatively minor revisions, for about 13 years.

2. General observations and comments about teaching and learning pharmacology in relation to nursing.

3. General teaching strategies that aim to promote student interest in and attention to drug therapy. The importance of drug therapy cannot be overemphasized because there are few areas of nursing with similar potentials for helping or harming clients.

4. Learning objectives, major chapter topics, a list of individual drugs, and teaching strategies for both classroom and clinical settings for each chapter of the text. The drug list consists mainly of prototypes and important or commonly used drugs (as indicated by the author's observations) and drugs often prescribed for outpatients. Teaching strategies for classroom use are cross-referenced to the text, *Study Guide,* and transparency masters in this manual to promote rapid retrieval and easier use. Any of these materials can be revised to meet the needs of individual instructors.

5. Transparency masters are provided for selected chapter content, including many of the illustrations in the text.

To fulfill the second purpose, test bank questions are provided for each chapter of the text. These follow the NCLEX format. In addition, sample solutions of several case studies from the *Study Guide* are included to assist instructors in using the case studies for classroom discussion.

SAMPLE COURSE SYLLABUS

COURSE DESCRIPTION

Introduction to clinical drug therapy with emphasis on the knowledge and interventions needed to maximize therapeutic effects and prevent or minimize adverse effects of drugs. Major content areas include basic concepts of pharmacology, groups of therapeutic drugs, prototypes of drug groups, commonly prescribed individual drugs, drug effects on body tissues, human responses to drug therapy, and applying nursing process in relation to prescribed drug therapy regimens.

Faculty

REQUIRED TEXT(S)

Course Objectives: Upon completion of this course, the student will be able to:

1. Define/describe terms, concepts, and basic processes associated with drug therapy.

2. Use a systematic approach to studying drug therapy, with emphasis on therapeutic classifications and prototypical drugs.

3. Describe characteristics of major drug groups and selected individual drugs in terms of the following:
   a. mechanism(s) of action
   b. indications for use
   c. therapeutic effects
   d. common or serious adverse effects
   e. accurate administration
   f. essential client teaching

4. Identify client-related and drug-related factors that influence drug effects.

5. Apply all steps of the nursing process in the care of clients receiving one or more therapeutic drugs.

6. Discuss principles of therapy with major drug groups in relation to drug selection, dosage, route, and use in selected populations.

7. Discuss clinically significant drug-drug, drug-disease, and drug-nutrient interactions.

8. Identify major issues/concerns in drug therapy of children, pregnant women, and older adults.

Acquisition Editor: Margaret Zuccarini
Assistant Editor: Sara Lauber
Ancillary Editor: Doris S. Wray
Production Manager: Helen Ewan
Production Editor: Virginia Barishek
Production Service: Berliner, Inc.
Printer/Binder: Victor Graphics

Fifth edition

6 5 4 3 2 1

ISBN: 0-7817-1482-6

Instructor's Manual and Testbank to Accompany

CLINICAL DRUG
THERAPY

RATIONALES FOR NURSING PRACTICE

Fifth Edition

Anne Collins Abrams, RN, MSN (Associate Professor)
Department of Baccalaureate and Graduate Nursing
College of Allied Health and Nursing
Eastern Kentucky University
Richmond, Kentucky

Gail Ropelewski-Ryan, RN, MSN (Professor)
Nurse Education, Health, Physical Education and Recreation
Corning Community College
Corning, New York

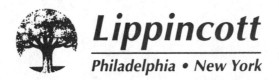

Lippincott
Philadelphia • New York

Contents

I

INTRODUCTION TO DRUG THERAPY

1
Introduction to Pharmacology

MAJOR TOPICS

Sources and names of drugs
Sources of drug information
Federal drug laws and standards; scheduled drugs
FDA drug-approval processes
Cellular physiology and response to injury
Chemical mediators of inflammation

OBJECTIVES

1. Differentiate between pharmacology and drug therapy.
2. Differentiate between generic and trade names of drugs.
3. Define a prototypical drug.
4. Select authoritative sources of drug information.
5. Differentiate the main categories of controlled substances in relation to therapeutic use and potential for abuse.
6. Discuss the role of the Food and Drug Administration.
7. Describe characteristics of normal cells in relation to drug therapy.
8. Describe cellular responses to injury, including inflammation.

TEACHING STRATEGIES

Classroom

1. Prepare and show a transparency of the 25 drugs most often prescribed for ambulatory clients (prepared from an annual list of the top 200 drugs dispensed in community pharmacies, usually published in the February or March issue of *American Druggist*). List the drugs by both generic and trade names. Ask students which they recognize, which they have given to clients, or which they have taken themselves.

2. Ask students to bring in a container of a prescription or OTC drug they've taken recently. List drug names on a transparency or marker board. Add therapeutic classifications or major indications for use and whether they will be studied in the course. The purpose of this exercise is to cre-

ate interest and motivation to learn about drug therapy, to emphasize that drug knowledge is relevant to personal lives as well as professional activities, and to emphasize that drug knowledge needs to be applied.

3. Show copies of various sources of drug information (e.g., textbooks, handbooks, *Physicians' Desk Reference*, *Drug Facts and Comparisons*, journal articles, and others) and discuss advantages and disadvantages of commonly used sources.

4. Provide a list of commonly used scheduled drugs. Ask students to designate the appropriate category of each drug and discuss nursing implications of administering the drug.

5. Show a transparency of Figure 1-1 (text, p. 213) to emphasize that body processes, including drug action, occur at the cellular level.

6. Discuss the role of selected chemical mediators (Box 1-2, text, pp. 8–9) in causing inflammation and that many drugs act to decrease the activity of one or more of these substances.

Clinical Laboratory

1. Have students identify scheduled drugs ordered for assigned clients.

2. Have each student select at least 2 drugs prescribed for an assigned client and consult a drug reference or make drug cards with important information. Course objective 3 (IM, p. v) can be used as an outline or format for content to be included. Encourage students to use their own words rather than copying the information. The mental processing required to restate the information aids learning and retention.

3. Have students look at a physician's order sheet for an assigned client and indicate whether drug names are generic or trade names.

4. Review with students the agency's policies related to scheduled drugs.

5. In a hospital setting, have one or more students list the scheduled drugs (from the medication administration record [MAR]) of several or all clients. This exercise will help students get a feel

for the extent of use in that unit and which individual drugs are more commonly used.

6. Ask students to identify signs and symptoms of inflammation observed in assigned clients.

7. Ask students to state examples of drugs used for systemic effects and drugs used for local effects.

TESTBANK QUESTIONS

1. J. is to administer furosemide. She realizes that this drug name is a:
   a. chemical name.
   b. trade name.
   c. official name.
   *d. generic name.

2. Naturally occurring substances that have been chemically modified are:
   a. synthetic compounds.
   *b. semisynthetic compounds.
   c. genetically engineered products.
   d. hybrid molecules.

3. Orphan drugs are:
   *a. used to treat uncommon disorders affecting relatively few people.
   b. used for investigational purposes.
   c. not regulated by the Food and Drug Administration.
   d. used in other countries but not approved in the United States.

4. During Phase II of drug trials, the investigational drug is administered to:
   a. animals.
   b. a large group of persons of various ages who are symptomatic.
   c. healthy volunteers.
   *d. a few subjects with the symptom or disease.

5. In the inflammatory process, histamine:
   a. releases oxidative metabolites.
   b. decreases vascular permeability.
   *c. causes vasodilation.
   d. engulfs pathogens.

6. A drug derived from a plant is:
   a. ether.
   b. iron.
   c. insulin.
   *d. morphine.

7. The Pure Food and Drug Act of 1906 contributes to medication safety by:
   a. regulating importation of narcotics.
   *b. establishing official drug standards and mandating labeling.
   c. mandating that synthetic drugs list adverse effects on the label.
   d. empowering states to enforce drug standards.

8. Drugs that come under Schedule V:
   a. are highly addictive.
   b. allow only 2 refills.
   *c. may be sold over the counter.
   d. require a prescription.

9. Assessment of a client receiving medication includes all of the following except:
   a. taking a personal and family history.
   b. obtaining information about allergies.
   c. obtaining a medical history, including over-the-counter medications.
   *d. modifying the physician's orders to accommodate the client's desires.

10. When administering oral medications to a client, you should:
    a. not give medications to a client with a naso-gastric tube in place.
    b. crush enteric coated tablets if the client has difficulty swallowing.
    c. administer cough medications first.
    *d. assess the client's ability to swallow.

2
Basic Concepts and Processes

MAJOR TOPICS

Mechanisms of drug movement
Pharmacokinetics—absorption, distribution, biotransformation, excretion
Pharmacodynamics—receptor theory of drug action at the cellular level
Drug-related variables that affect drug actions
Client-related variables that affect drug actions
Adverse drug reactions

OBJECTIVES

1. Describe the main mechanisms by which drugs cross biological membranes and move through the body.
2. Define each process of pharmacokinetics.
3. Describe drug-related factors that influence each pharmacokinetic process.
4. Describe client-related factors that influence each pharmacokinetic process.
5. Discuss drug actions at the cellular level (pharmacodynamics).
6. Describe major characteristics of the receptor theory of drug action.
7. Differentiate between agonist drugs and antagonist drugs.
8. Identify signs and symptoms that may occur with adverse drug effects on major body systems.

TEACHING STRATEGIES

Classroom

1. Lecture/discussion of pharmacokinetic processes and influencing factors:
   a. Define absorption and describe factors that increase or decrease absorption of an oral tablet or capsule (e.g., rate of dissolution in gastric fluids, GI-tract motility, presence of other drugs or foods in the GI tract, blood flow to the GI tract).
   b. Define distribution. Discuss the need for adequate cardiovascular function to maintain blood flow to body tissues. Show a transparency of Figure 2-1 (text, p. 13; IM, p. 126) and discuss the importance of adequate plasma proteins (e.g., serum albumin) to bind drug molecules. Emphasize that only free or unbound drug molecules can leave the bloodstream and act on body tissues.
   c. Define metabolism and biotransformation. Discuss the importance of adequate blood flow to the liver and factors that induce or inhibit drug-metabolizing enzymes in the liver.
   d. Define excretion and discuss the importance of kidney function in relation to eliminating drug molecules from the body.

2. Lecture/discussion of the receptor theory of drug action:
   a. Describe characteristics of receptors.
   b. Show a transparency of Figure 2-2 (text, p. 14; IM, p. 127).
   c. Emphasize similarities of many drugs to naturally occurring body substances.

3. Discuss selected variables that affect drug action (e.g., drug dosage, client's weight and health status).

4. Emphasize the need to actively assess clients for adverse drug reactions (ADRs) because ADRs may cause virtually any sign or symptom.

5. Show a transparency of major body systems affected by ADRs and ask students how they would recognize the ADRs (i.e., specific signs and symptoms) (IM, p. 128).

6. State a serum albumin level; ask if a client is at increased risk of ADRs. Ask students to state rationales for their answers.

Clinical Laboratory

1. Have students identify scheduled drugs ordered for assigned clients.

2. Ask students to assess assigned clients for GI, cardiovascular, hepatic, or renal disorders that can interfere with absorption, distribution, metabolism, or excretion of drugs.

3. Ask students to assess clients for at least one specific ADR that may occur with the client's prescribed drug therapy regimen.

4. Ask students to record laboratory reports (e.g., serum albumin levels, blood urea nitrogen, serum creatinine, AST, ALT), when available for an assigned client, and evaluate the client's risk for ADRs or drug-drug interactions.

TESTBANK QUESTIONS

1. When reviewing the product information available on a drug, the nurse finds that the drug is teratogenic. The nurse would know that this drug should not be administered to:
   a. asthmatic clients.
   *b. pregnant clients.
   c. children.
   d. clients with renal failure.

2. All the following types of medication preparations can produce local therapeutic effects *except* a(n):
   a. ointment.
   b. suppository.
   c. gel.
   *d. caplet.

3. A medication that enhances liver metabolism is referred to as a(n):
   *a. enzyme inducer.
   b. agonist.
   c. antagonist.
   d. synergist.

4. A medication is in a sustained-release tablet. The nurse should avoid:
   a. administering the tablet with another medication.
   b. giving the drug with an antacid.
   *c. crushing the tablet before administration.
   d. administering the tablet with water.

5. You know that the fastest and most effective route of administration for antibiotics is:
   a. oral.
   b. subcutaneous.
   *c. intravenous.
   d. intramuscular.

6. The advantage of sublingual administration of medication is that:
   a. first-pass effect occurs more quickly.
   b. it allows for slow dissolution and prolongs the effect.
   *c. drugs are not affected by GI secretions.
   d. the avascular portion of the lingual area is avoided.

7. The location for the metabolism of most medications is the:
   a. large intestine.
   *b. liver.
   c. pancreas.
   d. stomach.

8. 250 mg of a drug with a half life of 4 hours should be completely eliminated from the body in approximately
   a. 18 hrs.
   b. 12 hrs.
   *c. 24 hrs.
   d. 48 hrs.

9. The following is true regarding drug solubility.
   a. Aqueous solutions are absorbed more slowly than oil-based medications.
   b. Fat soluble drugs cannot cross the blood-brain barrier.
   c. Alcohol-based drugs are more slowly absorbed than oil-based drugs.
   *d. Nonionized drug forms are available for absorption.

10. The following is true regarding drug distribution.
    a. Most drugs in the serum are bound to hormones.
    *b. Adequate perfusion is necessary for drug distribution.
    c. Decreased cardiac output increases drug concentration.
    d. Drugs cross the placenta by active transport.

3
Administering Medications

MAJOR TOPICS

Five rights of drug administration
Medication orders/prescriptions
Drug preparations and dosage forms
Calculating drug dosages
Routes of administration
General techniques of drug administration

OBJECTIVES

1. List the five rights of drug administration.
2. Discuss knowledge and skills needed to implement the five rights.
3. List the requirements of a complete drug order or prescription.
4. Accurately interpret drug orders containing common abbreviations.
5. Discuss advantages and disadvantages of oral, parenteral, and topical routes of drug administration.
6. Identify supplies, techniques, and observations needed for safe, accurate administration by different routes.

TEACHING STRATEGIES

Classroom

1. Show a transparency of the five rights of drug administration and the requisite knowledge and skills (IM, p. 129).

2. Show a transparency of correct and incorrect drug orders and have students identify each. For incorrect orders, ask students to identify the part that is erroneous and to explain how to revise the order to make it correct.

3. List and discuss advantages and disadvantages of various routes of drug administration.

4. If not previously covered elsewhere, show equipment (e.g., oral and parenteral unit dose medications, needles, and syringes) and discuss criteria for selecting them.

5. Ask which specific equipment/site/technique would be appropriate for:
   a. an SC injection.
   b. an IM injection to an 8-month-old child, an obese adult, and a debilitated adult.
   c. administering a liquid and a pill via a nasogastric tube.

6. List types and examples of drugs that should not be crushed (e.g., enteric coated or long-acting tablets or capsules). These formulations are often labeled "extended release," "sustained action," or for once or twice daily administration. Note that various abbreviations are used and the drug name may not clearly indicate that it is a long-acting formulation.

7. Discuss the types of drugs often given PRN (e.g., analgesics, antiemetics) and the criteria the nurse may use to guide decision-making about administering PRN medications.

8. Discuss possible approaches to an adult client who refuses an important medication.

9. Discuss possible interventions when assessment of a client's condition seems to contraindicate a particular drug or a particular dose of a drug.

10. Discuss possible replies and actions when a client questions the number or types of medications being offered.

11. Discuss possible interventions when a student realizes he or she has given a medication to the wrong patient or made a medication error in relation to any of the five rights.

12. Discuss possible interventions when a student discovers that someone else has made a medication error in relation to any of the five rights.

13. Discuss possible interventions when a nurse or a student suspects a coworker of drug abuse.

14. Discuss safety factors related to drug administration to children and elderly adults, and in hospital and home settings.

Clinical Laboratory

1. Discuss a specific institution's policies and procedures regarding drug administration and recording.

2. In a hospital or long-term care facility, have students administer medications to their assigned clients, including alternative routes (e.g., NG tube, injections, inhalation, topically to skin).

3. Have students analyze assigned clients' medications for:
   a. drugs given for systemic effects.
   b. drugs given for local effects.
   c. non-oral dosage forms and routes of administration.
   d. tablets or capsules that should not be crushed.
   e. drugs that may be left at the bedside.
   f. drugs that may be self-administered by the client.
   g. type, frequency of administration, reason for use, and effects of PRN drugs.
   h. questions a client might ask about a drug and appropriate ways to answer them.

4. In an outpatient setting, have students ask clients about how they self-administer their medications and have students evaluate methods in relation to safe administration practices (for medications in general and for specific drugs the client is taking).

TESTBANK QUESTIONS

1. A Tylenol rectal suppository is ordered. You are aware that the medication is:
   a. inserted with its covering intact.
   *b. stored in the refrigerator.
   c. mixed with a gel before insertion.
   d. expelled within a minute after insertion.

2. Tetracycline 250 mg is ordered t.i.d. The best schedule to follow is:
   a. 9 a.m., 1 p.m., 5 p.m.
   b. 6 a.m., 12 p.m., 6 p.m.
   c. 8 a.m., 1 p.m., 6 p.m.
   *d. 7 a.m., 4 p.m., 11 p.m.

3. When administering medications, the nurse must do all of the following *except*:
   a. observing for therapeutic effects.
   b. instructing the client about the drug.
   c. checking the dose of the drug.
   *d. changing the dose if side effects occur.

4. The nurse administers an IV bolus of lidocaine to treat ventricular dysrhythmias. A bolus is a:
   a. continuous infusion given over a 24-hour period.
   *b. concentrated dose given over a short time period.
   c. slow infusion given over 1 hour.
   d. diluted dose given 1 to 6 times a day.

5. The physician writes an order: Garamycin gtt i in OS. You will administer the drug in the client's:
   a. left ear.
   b. right ear.
   *c. left eye.
   d. right eye.

6. Which statement is true regarding oral medication?
   a. Gastric upset is rare.
   *b. Aspiration can occur in seriously ill clients.
   c. When medication is given with water, absorption is decreased.
   d. Oral administration of medication is the fastest acting route.

7. All of the following are parenteral routes of administration *except:*
   *a. sublingual.
   b. intra-articular.
   c. subcutaneous.
   d. intrathecal.

8. When administering a narcotic analgesic intramuscularly, the nurse should:
   a. inject the medication as quickly as possible.
   b. insert and remove the needle very slowly and carefully.
   *c. calm the client by talking to him or her.
   d. inject the medication into a tightened muscle.

4
Nursing Process in Drug Therapy

MAJOR TOPICS

Legal responsibilities of the nurse
Applying the nursing process in drug therapy—assessment, nursing diagnosis, planning/goals, interventions (including teaching), and evaluation
General principles of drug therapy—goals, benefits versus risks, individualization, drug selection, drug use in children and older adults

OBJECTIVES

1. Develop personal techniques for learning and using drug knowledge in client care.
2. Assess clients' conditions in relation to age, weight, health-illness status (especially renal and cardiovascular functions), lifestyle habits likely to influence drug effects, and use of OTC and prescription drugs.
3. Obtain a medication history.
4. Identify nondrug interventions to prevent or decrease the need for drug therapy.
5. Discuss interventions to increase benefits and decrease hazards of drug therapy.
6. Discuss guidelines for rational choices of drugs, dosages, routes, and times of administration.

7. Observe clients for therapeutic and adverse responses to drug therapy.
8. Teach clients and family members safe and effective drug administration.
9. Discuss application of the nursing process in home care settings.
10. Discuss legal, ethical, and economic implications of drug therapy.

TEACHING STRATEGIES

Classroom

1. Emphasize that students already know the steps of the nursing process; now they need to apply those steps in drug therapy.

2. Show a transparency of the medication history (text, p. 40) and discuss the rationale for obtaining the designated information. Emphasize that the information can readily be incorporated into any assessment tool and that a separate medication history is not required.

3. Ask students to identify additional sources of drug-related information, including various textbooks and a client's medical records.

4. Demonstrate ways to analyze assessment data to determine the client's nursing care needs related to drug therapy (e.g., implications related to the client's age and medical diagnoses, as well as the prescribed drugs).

5. Ask students to identify laboratory tests that help to assess a client's response to drug therapy (therapeutic or adverse).

6. Provide assessment information and a list of drugs ordered for a client; assign small groups to write a nursing care plan (nursing diagnosis, goals, interventions, evaluation criteria).

7. Emphasize that students already know principles of teaching/learning; now they need to apply the principles in relation to drug therapy. They also need to consider the client's education and reading level.

8. Discuss information a client usually needs about a newly prescribed drug and resources and methodologies for providing this information.

9. For a client who has been taking a drug for a while, discuss assessment of learning needs in relation to the drug. Ask students to state specific questions to assess a client's knowledge and medication-taking behavior.

10. For a client started on a new drug while hospitalized, discuss factors to be considered in discharge teaching about the drug. How does the new drug fit with the client's other drugs (if any)? Are there activity or dietary restrictions needed with the new drug? What if the patient is a child or an elderly adult?

11. Divide the class into small groups and name a commonly used drug (one likely to be familiar to some students). Assign half of the groups to discuss #9 and half to discuss #10. Have one or two groups from each half to share their findings with the whole class.

12. Provide a client care situation and ask individual students (out of class) or small groups (in class) to write a teaching plan for at least two medications. Some guidelines are provided in the "Teaching Plan for Medications" below.

13. Provide a copy of an instruction sheet dispensed with an outpatient prescription drug. Have students critique it for usefulness for an individual patient and individualize it for that patient (actual or hypothetical).

14. Obtain a copy of an agency clinical pathway and transfer it to a transparency to demonstrate the relationship of drug therapy to other elements.

15. Provide a copy of or information from an OTC drug label and have students critique it for use by themselves or most patients.

16. Discuss costs of medications—a list of costs of commonly used drugs can be obtained from a pharmacy (sometimes the *Medical Letter on Drugs and Therapeutics* publishes a list of costs, usually when a new drug is approved, such as a new NSAID or antibiotic) or the instructor and students can share their experiences and personal purchases.

Clinical Laboratory

1. For an assigned client, have students complete a medication history, obtain additional assessment data from the client's medical records, analyze data with the help of appropriate references and textbooks, and write a nursing care plan that reflects the client's needs related to drug therapy.

2. Have students do initial and discharge teaching of clients when the opportunity arises.

3. Given two patients receiving the same drug, ask students to compare and contrast assessment data (including whether the drug is newly prescribed or long-term) in relation to important information about the drug and compare and contrast the teaching/learning needs of the two clients. This exercise will help reinforce the principle that all drug therapy should be individualized.

4. For clients at home, have students review the drugs being taken and provide clients an opportunity to ask questions, state concerns, and identify any difficulties they've encountered with the medications.

Teaching Plan for Medications

1. For a "general" teaching plan related to a particular drug, include information likely to be helpful to most people for whom the drug is prescribed.

2. For a specific client, consider client-related factors (e.g., age, medical diagnosis, laboratory and other diagnostic test reports, nursing database, medication history) and drug-related information (e.g., type of drug, indications for use, adverse effects) to assess the client's learning needs about a particular drug. More specifically, try to determine the following:
   a. What does the client already know?
   b. What does the client need to know?
   c. What does the client want to know?

3. Write specific, measurable, attainable objectives. (Use action verbs such as list, write, verbalize, and state rather than know or understand, for example.)

4. List content to be covered. (With a newly prescribed drug, most of the information listed below will be needed. With a drug the client has been taking for a while, specific content is determined by the client's knowledge about the drug and the nurse's assessment data about the client's compliance, therapeutic and adverse responses, and other individualized information.)
   a. Name of drug.
   b. Reason for use (what it will do for the client in terms of relieving symptoms, preventing problems, etc.).
   c. Prescribing information (dose, frequency of administration, etc.).
   d. Adverse effects to be reported.
   e. Preparation or storage instructions, if indicated.

5. List methods of instruction, including verbal, written (self or booklets), and audiovisual aids.

6. To evaluate teaching, state criteria indicating whether objective was met or not met.

7. Use four columns with the headings of Objectives, Content, Methods of Instruction, and Evaluation.

TESTBANK QUESTIONS

1. You are administering erythromycin to 3-year-old J. Before administering medication to J., you should:
   a. ask him to state his name.
   b. dilute the medication with juice and put it in a syringe.
   c. place him in a highchair.
   *d. determine if the dose is appropriate.

2. Which of the following statements by 93-year-old Mrs. S. leads you to believe that she may have a problem with over-the-counter medications?
   a. "I take Metamucil every night before I go to sleep."
   b. "I take a vitamin pill every morning with my breakfast."
   c. "I use aspirin when I have a headache."
   *d. "I use sodium bicarbonate before each meal to prevent heartburn."

3. You are to administer morphine intravenously to an 89-year-old client with impaired hepatic function. You should be aware that this will:
   a. increase the dose required.
   *b. increase the risk of drug toxicity.
   c. limit the times the medication can be given.
   d. decrease elimination of the drug.

4. A 76-year-old diabetic is being admitted for repair of a fractured hip. Which of the following questions would be most helpful in eliciting information for an admission nursing assessment?
   a. "You do not have problems with giving yourself insulin, do you?"
   b. "Who told you you could use honey in your tea?"
   *c. "What do you do if you become shaky?"
   d. "Do you take daily laxatives?"

5. A client tells you about an allergic reaction to a medication. Which of the following would be indicative of an allergic reaction?
   *a. Rash
   b. Nausea
   c. Dizziness
   d. Drowsiness

6. Which of the following statements by a client receiving Coumadin indicates that health teaching regarding the medication has been ineffective?
   a. "I love chocolate candy and eat it several times a week."
   b. "I ate a chocolate candy bar yesterday."
   *c. "I always have a bottle of aspirin with me."
   d. "I use a laxative every other day."

7. Which statement by a client receiving a medication would indicate that health teaching was ineffective?
   a. "I have had trouble taking medicine on time."
   b. "My father had Parkinson's disease and he lived a long time."
   *c. "Missing a pill now and then doesn't matter."
   d. "Medication is usually more rapid-acting when taken on an empty stomach."

8. The following would be an appropriate outcome for clients receiving medications. The client will:
   *a. state the reasons for taking the medicine.
   b. know how the medication works.
   c. understand why he must watch for side effects.
   d. understand the disease process.

9. It is important to gather information about a client receiving antiparkinson medications. All of the following are examples of subjective data gathered during the admission process *except:*
    a. dietary modifications.
    b. perceptions about illness.
    c. ways of coping.
    *d. gait disturbances.

10. When taking a medication history, you know:
    a. heavy smoking has no impact on medication action.
    b. alcohol decreases the action of CNS drugs.
    c. over-the-counter drugs do not need to be included.
    *d. clients allergic to fish may also be allergic to contrast dye.

11. The following is true regarding the planning stage of the nursing process.
    *a. Goals are the outcomes that are evaluated.
    b. The client is not involved initially in the planning of care.
    c. Compliance does not depend upon a client's acceptance of a diagnosis.
    d. Nursing diagnoses are based solely on the subjective assessment.

CRITICAL THINKING CASE STUDY

M. weighs 44 lbs. or 20 kilograms.

1. If the recommended dosage range of phenobarbital is 4–6 mg/kg/day, then the maximum daily dose should be 120 mg a day.

2. If the medication is administered in 3 equal dosages, M. should receive 40 mg per dose.

3. Phenobarbital comes in 15 mg/ml. You should administer 2.66 ml or 2.7 ml.

4. The minimum dose of Dilantin is 80 mg per day or 40 mg b.i.d.

5. The maximum dose of Dilantin is 140 mg per day or 70 mg b.i.d.

6. If you are administering the minimum dose of 40 mg per dose, you would give 1.33 ml. If you are administering the maximum dose of 70 mg per dose, you would give 1.4 ml.

7. The medication could be administered in the abdomen, thigh, arm.

8. The maximum dose for M. should be 4 mg. The order exceeds the maximum dose, therefore the nurse should speak with the physician.

II
DRUGS AFFECTING THE CENTRAL NERVOUS SYSTEM

5
Physiology of the Central Nervous System

MAJOR TOPICS

Characteristics and functions of the CNS, including neurotransmitters
Characteristics of CNS depression and stimulation

OBJECTIVES

1. Describe the process of neurotransmission.
2. Describe major neurotransmitters and their roles in nervous system functioning.
3. Discuss signs and symptoms of CNS depression.
4. Discuss general types and characteristics of CNS depressant drugs.

TEACHING STRATEGIES

Classroom

1. Assign chapter to be read—before discussion of antianxiety, antipsychotic, and antidepressant medications. Information about neurotransmitters, receptors, and so on is essential to understanding clinical effects of these drugs.

2. Discuss CNS neurotransmission systems.

3. Show a transparency of Figure 5-1 (text, p. 55; IM, p. 131).

4. Discuss common disorders associated with deficiency or excess of particular neurotransmitters.

5. Discuss drug actions that mimic or block actions of naturally occurring neurotransmitters.

6. Discuss review and application exercises 7 and 8 (text, p. 60).

Clinical Laboratory

1. Have students assess each assigned client in terms of level of consciousness and overt mental health status.

2. For assigned clients, ask students to identify those with either disease processes or drug thera-py regimens associated with altered neurotransmitter functions.

TESTBANK QUESTIONS

1. Mr. C., who suffered a head injury this morning, has an elevated temperature that is difficult to control with antipyretics. This is a result of swelling around his:
   a. thalamus.
   b. cerebrum.
   c. pituitary.
   *d. hypothalamus.

2. When administering morphine, the nurse must assess:
   a. peripheral pulses.
   b. heart sounds.
   c. bowel sounds.
   *d. respiratory rate.

3. Mr. J., who is admitted for a myocardial infarction, is started on nitroglycerin. His blood pressure drops; this is due to:
   a. stimulation of the hypothalamus.
   b. pain associated with the infarction.
   *c. vasodilation.
   d. central nervous system depression.

4. The following is a neurotransmitter:
   a. Calcium ion
   b. Cholinesterase
   *c. Serotonin
   d. Monamine oxidase

5. Hypoxia:
   a. increases synaptic transmission.
   *b. causes CNS depression.
   c. alters neurotransmitter synthesis.
   d. results in neurotransmitter degradation.

6. The following are receptors embedded in the cell membranes of neurons:
   *a. Proteins
   b. Hormones
   c. Enzymes
   d. Ions

7. Synaptic transmission is decreased as a result of:
   a. hypokalemia.
   *b. acidosis.
   c. hypocalcemia.
   d. alkalosis.

8. This neurotransmitter is associated with the level of arousal, memory, and speech:
   a. Dopamine
   *b. Acetylcholine
   c. Gamma-aminobutyric acid
   d. Norepinephrine

9. A decrease in the following neurotransmitter substance is associated with Huntington's disease:
   a. Acetylcholine
   b. Dopamine
   *c. Glutamate
   d. Serotonin

10. The hypothalamus:
    a. relays motor impulses from the cortex to the spinal cord.
    b. is responsible for voluntary movement.
    *c. continually adjusts body temperature, blood pressure, and heart rate.
    d. helps maintain red blood cell production.

11. ADH secretion is controlled by:
    *a. the osmolarity of the extracellular fluid.
    b. cardiac output.
    c. the kidneys.
    d. the pH of body fluids.

12. Reflex centers for coughing, vomiting, sneezing, and swallowing are located in the:
    a. reticular activating system.
    b. limbic system.
    c. pons.
    *d. medulla oblongata.

13. A thiamine deficiency can cause:
    *a. degeneration of the myelin sheaths of nerve cells.
    b. mental confusion and dizziness.
    c. involuntary reflexes.
    d. hyperactivity, nervousness, and insomnia.

14. When administering CNS depressants, you should assess:
    a. peripheral pulses.
    b. heart sounds.
    c. bowel sounds.
    *d. respiratory rate.

6
Narcotic Analgesics and Narcotic Antagonists

MAJOR TOPICS

Pain
Description of narcotic analgesics
Classifications and individual drugs
Nursing process in relation to pain assessment and management
Principles of therapy

DRUG LIST

Codeine
Meperidine (Demerol)
Morphine sulfate
Naloxone (Narcan)
Tramadol (Ultram)

Acetaminophen/narcotic combinations
Acetaminophen with codeine (e.g., Tylenol #3)
Hydrocodone/APAP (e.g., Hydrocet, Lorcet, Lortab, Vicodin)
Oxycodone/acetaminophen (e.g., Percocet, Roxicet, Tylox)

OBJECTIVES

1. Discuss characteristics of pain.
2. Discuss the nurse's role in managing clients' pain.
3. List characteristics of narcotic analgesics in terms of mechanism of action, indications for use, and major adverse effects.
4. Describe morphine as the prototype of narcotic analgesics.
5. Discuss morphine dosage forms and dosage ranges for various clinical uses.
6. Explain why higher doses of narcotic analgesics are needed when the drugs are given orally.
7. Contrast the use of narcotic analgesics in "opiate-naive" and "opiate-tolerant" clients.
8. Assess the level of consciousness and respiratory status before and after administering narcotics.
9. Discuss principles of therapy and nursing process for using narcotic analgesics in children and older adults.
10. Teach clients about safe, effective use of narcotic analgesics.
11. Discuss the clinical use of narcotic antagonists.

TEACHING STRATEGIES

Classroom

1. Compare and contrast acute pain and chronic pain.

2. Discuss nursing assessment of pain, including whether pain is objective (a sign) or subjective (a symptom).

3. Describe or demonstrate various pain assessment scales and tools.

4. Discuss interventions to prevent pain and non-pharmacologic methods of relieving pain.

5. Lecture/discussion about morphine as the prototype narcotic analgesic in terms of mechanism of action, indications for use, therapeutic effects, common or serious adverse effects, accurate administration, and essential client/family teaching.

6. Ask students about factors the nurse should consider in deciding whether to give or not give a PRN narcotic analgesic. Write factors on a transparency or marker board. Put an asterisk or checkmark by those factors with a high degree of consensus; discuss factors with low consensus further.

7. Discuss the nursing care of a client receiving an intravenous (by continuous infusion or PCA pump) or epidural narcotic analgesic.

8. Ask students to share their experiences with pain and their various methods of relieving pain.

9. Outline treatment measures for narcotic overdose, including indications for use and expected effects of a narcotic antagonist.

10. Discuss pain management as a component of perioperative care.

11. Compare and contrast narcotic and non-narcotic analgesics in terms of effectiveness and adverse effects.

12. Discuss the rationale for combining narcotic and non-narcotic analgesics.

13. Compare the nursing implications of administering strong parenteral narcotics and oral narcotic/non-narcotic combination drugs.

14. Assign small groups to complete the Critical Thinking Case Study (SG, p. 25), then discuss as a class.

15. For a home-care client, discuss ways to increase the safety of narcotic analgesic administration.

Clinical Laboratory

1. For a client receiving a narcotic analgesic, have a student assess the level of consciousness, respiratory status, and other safety factors and verbalize at least one nursing diagnosis relevant to the drug therapy.

2. Assign a student to assess a client's need for a pain medication, administer a narcotic analgesic, and evaluate the client's response about 30 minutes after drug administration.

3. Ask a patient with a PCA pump or epidural narcotic analgesic for permission to show the device to students who have not previously seen it. Include the patient in any demonstration or discussion that occurs at the bedside. Interview the client regarding effectiveness of the method in managing pain and any difficulties experienced with it.

4. Have students list the narcotic/non-narcotic analgesics (e.g., generic and trade names and amounts of each ingredient) that are commonly used in the clinical agency.

5. Discuss morphine dosage forms and dosage ranges for various clinical uses.

TESTBANK QUESTIONS

1. The physician orders 5 mg of morphine (Roxanol) q2h. Roxanol contains 20 mg/ml. How many drops will you administer?
   a. 2 gtts
   *b. 4 gtts
   c. 6 gtts
   d. 8 gtts

2. Mrs. G., who has a PCA pump, states, "I'm afraid to use this device. I'm worried that I will give myself too much medication." Identify the *best* response.
   a. The doctor would never order a PCA pump for you if he thought that could happen.
   b. If you follow the directions that you have been given, that will not happen.
   c. The PCA device always provides the correct amount, never too much, never too little.
   *d. The device is preset, and therefore you can only receive a specific amount every few minutes.

3. Your client has been taking morphine q4h for back pain. It is important to assess him for:
   a. diarrhea.
   *b. constipation.
   c. cough.
   d. urinary frequency.

4. The following analgesic is commonly given with acetaminophen (Tylenol) for moderate pain:
   *a. Codeine
   b. Phenergan
   c. Advil
   d. Talwin

5. The following drug could be used to reverse the effects of morphine:
   *a. Naloxone hydrochloride (Narcan)
   b. Butorphanol tartrate (Stadol)
   c. Buprenorphine (Buprenex)
   d. Nalbuphine hydrochloride (Nubain)

6. The following is attributable to long-term administration of narcotics:
   a. Tachycardia
   b. Decreased pain perception
   c. Irritable bowel syndrome
   *d. Tolerance

7. An adverse effect of the administration of narcotics is:
   *a. hypotension.
   b. hyperkalemia.
   c. dry mouth.
   d. blurred vision.

8. Opiates should not be administered to clients with head injuries because they decrease:
   *a. pupillary response.
   b. urinary output.
   c. core body temperature.
   d. peripheral vasodilation.

9. The nurse should be aware that a common adverse reaction of intravenous morphine is:
   a. bronchial constriction.
   b. hypoxia.
   *c. respiratory depression.
   d. stasis of secretions.

10. The following analgesic should be administered to the client who has had a craniotomy:
   *a. Acetaminophen with codeine (Tylenol with codeine)
   b. Propoxyphene hydrochloride (Darvon)
   c. Levorphanol tartrate (Levo-Dromoran)
   d. Morphine sulfate (Roxanol)

CRITICAL THINKING CASE STUDY

1. "It is necessary to begin to decrease your pain medication so that you do not become dependent upon it. We will wean you gradually off the medication while we increase your activity and that should control your pain."

2. Constipation is a common adverse effect of administration of narcotic analgesics. Daily documentation of bowel patterns, increased mobility, roughage, and fluid intake should help to minimize constipation.

3. You should start by finding out the location and extent of pain that M.G. was experiencing. You need to document the teaching that you did with M.G. in the morning. Your plan for weaning M.G. off the pain medication needs to be discussed with the other staff members and included in the plan of care. M.G. also needs additional teaching.

7
Analgesic–Antipyretic–Anti-inflammatory and Related Drugs

MAJOR TOPICS

Prostaglandins and their effects
Characteristics of aspirin and NSAIDs
Nursing process and principles of therapy related to clients with fever, pain, inflammation, gout, and migraine

DRUG LIST

Acetaminophen (Tylenol, others)
Acetylcysteine (Mucomyst)
Aspirin
Diclofenac (Voltaren)
Etodolac (Lodine)
Ibuprofen (Motrin, Advil, others)
Ketoprofen (Orudis, Oruvail)
Naproxen (Naprosyn, Aleve)
Nabumetone (Relafen)
Oxaprozin (Daypro)
Sumatriptan (Imitrex)

OBJECTIVES

1. Discuss the role of prostaglandins in the etiology of pain, fever, and inflammation.
2. Discuss aspirin and selected other nonsteroidal anti-inflammatory drugs (NSAIDs) in terms of mechanism of action, indications for use, nursing process, administration, and principles of therapy.
3. Compare and contrast aspirin, acetaminophen, and ibuprofen (Motrin) in terms of indications for use and adverse effects.
4. Differentiate among anti-platelet, analgesic, and anti-inflammatory doses of aspirin.
5. Teach clients interventions to prevent or decrease adverse effects of aspirin, other NSAIDs, and acetaminophen.
6. Identify factors influencing the use of aspirin, NSAIDs, and acetaminophen in children and older adults.
7. Discuss the use of acetylcysteine as an antidote for acetaminophen overdose.
8. Discuss nursing implications of drug therapy for gout and migraine.

TEACHING STRATEGIES

Classroom

1. Show a transparency of Table 7-1 (text, p. 79; IM, p. 132) and discuss antiprostaglandin effects of aspirin and related drugs.
2. Ask about students' experiences with aspirin, acetaminophen, and ibuprofen (e.g., personal preference and why, conditions drugs were used for, what kind of results were obtained, and whether they used generic or trade formulations).
3. Show a transparency of indications for use (Table 7-2, text, p. 81; IM, p. 133).
4. Ask students to compare and contrast aspirin, acetaminophen, and ibuprofen in terms of indications for use and adverse effects. In addition to ibuprofen, diclofenac, etodolac, ketoprofen, naproxen, nabumetone, and oxaprozin are commonly used NSAIDs; ketoprofen and naproxen are also available OTC. The instructor may wish to compare the other drugs to ibuprofen and perhaps add ketorolac (Toradol) to the drug list, because students are likely to encounter any of the drugs in multiple clinical settings.

5. Given a client with a nursing diagnosis of Risk for Injury related to aspirin or NSAID-induced gastric ulceration and GI bleeding, have students identify or write nursing interventions to reduce risk.

6. Discuss major elements of treating overdoses of aspirin and acetaminophen.

7. Discuss review and application exercises 4, 5, and 6 (text, p. 93) regarding drug selection for a child, a middle-aged adult, and an elderly adult.

8. Assign small groups to complete the Critical Thinking Case Study (SG, p. 27), then discuss as a class.

Clinical Laboratory

1. For clients receiving aspirin or an NSAID, have students assess for knowledge about safe usage and risk for adverse effects.

2. For clients receiving aspirin or an NSAID, have students question them about the occurrence of adverse drug effects.

3. For clients receiving aspirin or an NSAID, have students prepare a teaching plan and include OTC sources of the same or a similar drug.

4. Given a client who takes OTC preparations of aspirin, acetaminophen, or ibuprofen, have students instruct client to read labels and follow instructions to ensure optimal therapeutic effects and minimize adverse effects.

5. During home visits, have students assess ages, health status, and use of prescription or OTC NSAIDs for all members of the household. Intervene when indicated.

TESTBANK QUESTIONS

1. Your client is started on allopurinol (Zyloprim) for gouty arthritis. He should be instructed to immediately report which of the following adverse effects?
   a. Headache and nausea
   *b. Unusual bruising
   c. Dry flaky skin
   d. Constipation or cramping

2. You should assess T., admitted with chronic ergot poisoning, for:
   a. blurred vision.
   b. tinnitus.
   c. hematuria.
   *d. hypertension.

3. Which of the following, if taken concurrently with aspirin, will decrease its effects?
   a. Acetaminophen
   *b. Maalox
   c. Caffeine
   d. Laxatives

4. A client taking ergotamine tartrate and caffeine (Cafergot) for migraine headaches should be instructed to:
   *a. take two tablets at the onset of a migraine, than 1 tablet every half hour; do not exceed 6 tablets per attack.
   b. take 1 tablet every 4 hours; if you still have a headache, use aspirin in between.
   c. lie down first; if your headache does not go away then take 2 tablets.
   d. not eat or drink anything for 4 hours after taking this medication.

5. Which of the following statements by a client taking naproxen (Naprosyn) for arthritis leads you to believe that she has understood the teaching you have done?
   a. "I will take the medication only after I have tried other remedies."
   b. "After taking the medication, I should get relief of pain within 5 to 10 minutes."
   *c. "I will avoid over the counter medications while I am using the drug."
   d. "If I think that there is a possibility I might have pain, I will take the medication."

6. The following medication is used for the treatment of an acute attack of gout:
   a. Sumatriptan (Imitrex)
   *b. Colchicine
   c. Hydroxychloroquine (Plaquenil)
   d. Cyclophosphamide (Cytoxan)

7. Which of the following adverse effects should a client receiving ibuprofen (Motrin, Advil) be instructed to report?
   *a. Melena
   b. Blurred vision
   c. Fever
   d. Headache

8. Which of the following medications, if administered concurrently with aspirin, will result in an additive effect?
   *a. Codeine
   b. Sodium bicarbonate
   c. Thiazide diuretics
   d. Caffeine

9. A 79 year old with renal insufficiency is started on indomethacin (Idocin). Which of the following assessments should be done on a regular basis?
   a. Serum chloride levels
   *b. Serum creatinine levels
   c. Breath sounds
   d. Blood glucose levels

10. A client admitted with a Tylenol overdose should be assessed for increased:
    a. creatinine levels.
    b. blood glucose levels.
    *c. SGOT/AST levels.
    d. uric acid levels.

11. A client admitted with acute acetaminophen (Tylenol) poisoning should be assessed for:
    a. respiratory depression.
    b. renal failure.
    *c. liver dysfunction.
    d. dysrhythmias.

12. Gold is used to treat:
    *a. arthritis.
    b. bursitis.
    c. dysmenorrhea.
    d. gout.

13. Which of the following analgesics is effective in the treatment of bursitis, tendinitis, and gout?
    a. Piroxicam (Feldene)
    *b. Aspirin
    c. Tolmetin (Tolectin)
    d. Acetaminophen (Tylenol)

14. The following drug decreases uric acid levels:
    *a. Allopurinol (Zyloprim)
    b. Acetaminophen (Tylenol)
    c. Ergotamine tartrate (Ergomar)
    d. Methysergide maleate (Sansert)

CRITICAL THINKING CASE STUDY

1. Uncommon but potential adverse effects related to Clinoril include gastrointestinal ulceration, hemolytic anemia, confusion, depression, and psychosis. The physician should be made aware of Mrs. J.'s past history of anemia and psychosis.

2. The periodic assessment would include a CBC to assess for anemia and bone marrow depression.

3. The nurse should teach Mrs. J. to avoid over the counter medications, avoid overuse of medications, institute treatment as soon as it is indicated, and utilize other measures instead of or along with drug therapy.

4. Ketorolac is effective for the treatment of severe pain associated with arthritis and reportedly causes less gastric irritation than Clinoril. This medication can also be given by injection and is reportedly comparable to morphine in its analgesic effectiveness.

8
Antianxiety and Sedative-Hypnotic Drugs

MAJOR TOPICS

Anxiety
Barbiturates
Benzodiazepines
Benzodiazepine receptors
Gamma-aminobutyric acid (GABA) as an inhibitory neurotransmitter
Insomnia
Sleep patterns and disorders

DRUG LIST

Alprazolam (Xanax)
Buspirone (BuSpar)
Diazepam (Valium)
Flumazenil (Romazicon)
Lorazepam (Ativan)
Temazepam (Restoril)
Zolpidem (Ambien)

OBJECTIVES

1. Discuss functions of sleep and consequences of sleep deprivation.
2. Discuss functions of sleep and consequences of anxiety.
3. Describe nondrug interventions to decrease anxiety and insomnia.
4. List characteristics of benzodiazepine antianxiety and hypnotic drugs in terms of mechanism of action, indications for use, nursing process implications, and potential for abuse and dependence.
5. Describe strategies for preventing, recognizing, or treating benzodiazepine withdrawal reactions.
6. Discuss characteristics of nonbenzodiazepine antianxiety and hypnotic agents.
7. Describe guidelines for rational, safe use of antianxiety and sedative-hypnotic drugs.
8. Discuss the use of flumazenil (Romazicon) and other treatment measures for overdose of benzodiazepines.

TEACHING STRATEGIES

Classroom

1. Ask students if sleep is necessary for health.
2. Ask students to describe how they feel when they've had enough sleep in comparison to the way they feel when sleep deprived.
3. Discuss consequences or potential hazards of sleep deprivation.
4. Discuss various terms a client might use to describe anxiety.
5. Discuss appearances and behaviors that might indicate anxiety.
6. Ask students how they feel when anxious and what they do to relieve anxiety.
7. List "sleep hygiene" factors that anyone can use to develop healthful sleep habits.
8. Give students about 5 minutes to write a list of nonpharmacologic interventions to decrease anxiety and insomnia, then discuss as a group.
9. Discuss the benefits of nonpharmacologic versus pharmacologic treatment of anxiety.
10. Show a transparency of antianxiety benzodiazepines (IM, p. 134).

11. Show a transparency of hypnotic benzodi-azepines (IM, p. 135).

12. Identify drugs that are likely to cause residual effects ("morning hangover") and impair daytime psychomotor performance.

13. Discuss client behaviors and verbal statements that may indicate a likelihood of compliance or abuse with prescribed hypnotic drugs.

14. Discuss the importance of teaching clients not to stop a benzodiazepine abruptly if it has been taken more than a few days.

15. Discuss review and application exercises 4, 8, 11, and 12 (text, pp. 108–109).

Clinical Laboratory

1. When observing behaviors that may indicate anxiety, interview the client when possible to validate feelings of anxiety. The instructor or a student may conduct the interview.

2. For an outpatient who takes an antianxiety or sedative-hypnotic drug, ask a student to teach safety measures, including listing other drugs that increase sedative effects.

3. For a client receiving an antianxiety or sedative-hypnotic drug, identify behaviors or verbal statements that may indicate a risk of overuse or abuse of the drug.

4. For a client with a nursing diagnosis of Sleep Pattern Disturbance: Insomnia, assign a student to assess for lifestyle and environmental etiologic factors and list interventions appropriate to the client and assessment data.

5. For a client with a nursing diagnosis of Knowledge Deficit with regard to nondrug measures for relieving stress and anxiety, have a student lead a post-conference group discussion about appropriate interventions.

6. For a hospitalized client with a nursing diagnosis of Risk for Injury related to sedation and other adverse effects, have a student lead a post-conference group discussion about interventions to protect the client.

7. In any clinical setting, have a student determine the location of (or the procedure for obtaining) flumazenil and report to the entire clinical group.

TESTBANK QUESTIONS

1. Problems associated with the use of barbiturates include:
   a. impairment of short-term memory.
   *b. induction of drug metabolizing enzymes in the liver.
   c. increase in REM sleep.
   d. enhancement of renal excretion of drugs.

2. Most sedative hypnotics lose their effectiveness with daily use in approximately:
   *a. 2 weeks.
   b. 1 month.
   c. 2 months.
   d. 1 year.

3. Compared to barbiturates, benzodiazepines do not:
   a. produce physiologic dependence or withdrawal symptoms.
   *b. suppress REM sleep.
   c. cause sedation.
   d. precipitate respiratory depression.

4. The length of time required before a client taking a benzodiazepine reaches a steady state is:
   a. 24 hours.
   b. 48 hours.
   c. 2 to 3 days.
   *d. 5 to 7 days.

5. Buspirone varies from other antianxiety drugs in that it:
   a. has muscle relaxant effects.
   b. has anticonvulsant effects.
   *c. does not cause physical or psychological dependence.
   d. causes CNS depression.

6. Hydroxyzine (Vistaril) is used preoperatively to minimize the following symptoms associated with surgery:
   *a. Anxiety, nausea, and vomiting
   b. Respiratory secretions
   c. Hypertension and tachycardia
   d. Depression

7. A hypnotic that reportedly does not suppress REM sleep is:
   a. pentobarbital (Nembutal).
   *b. chloral hydrate.
   c. flurazepam (Dalmane).
   d. amobarbital sodium (Amytal).

8. Sedative hypnotics are contraindicated for persons with the following disorder(s):
   a. Neurological diseases
   *b. Liver failure
   c. Endocrine disorders
   d. Heart disease

9. A Symptom of insomnia that the nurse should assess for prior to the administration of hypnotics is:
   a. agitation.
   *b. difficulty concentrating.
   c. anorexia.
   d. increased muscle tension.

10. An antidote for benzodiazepine toxicity is:
    *a. flumazenil (Romazicon).
    b. clomipramine (Anafranil).
    c. hydroxyzine (Vistaril).
    d. zolpidem (Ambien).

11. You know that your teaching has been effective if a client who is taking benzodiazepines states:
    a. "I will only take the medication at bedtime."
    *b. "I will not discontinue the medication abruptly."
    c. "I cannot take this medication if I am using pain medication."
    d. "I will need this medication the rest of my life."

12. Concurrent administration of the following drug with antianxiety agents will decrease their effects:
    a. Calcium
    *b. Caffeine
    c. Alcohol
    d. Aspirin

9
Antipsychotic Drugs

MAJOR TOPICS
Schizophrenia as a major psychotic disorder
Neurotransmission systems in psychosis

DRUG LIST
Chlorpromazine (Thorazine)
Clozapine (Clozaril)
Haloperidol (Haldol)
Olanzapine (Zyprexa)
Risperidone (Risperdal)

OBJECTIVES
1. Discuss schizophrenia and common manifestations of psychotic disorders.
2. Discuss characteristics of phenothiazines and related antipsychotics in terms of mechanism of action, indications for use, adverse effects, principles of therapy, and nursing process implications.
3. Compare characteristics of clozapine, risperidone, and olanzapine with those of phenothiazines and related antipsychotic drugs.
4. State interventions to promote compliance with outpatient use of antipsychotic drugs.

TEACHING STRATEGIES

Classroom
1. Ask students what verbal and nonverbal behaviors would make them suspect psychosis.

2. Discuss phenothiazines and related drugs as the prototypical drugs, and discuss risperidone as a commonly used drug.

3. Discuss possible approaches to promote compliance with the prescribed antipsychotic drug therapy regimen.

4. For outpatients, discuss the importance of teaching a family member or caretaker about drug therapy.

5. Discuss specific appearances and behaviors that may indicate adverse effects of antipsychotic drugs, and list interventions for minimizing each adverse effect.

6. For clients in hospitals or long-term care facilities who become agitated, noisy, and disruptive, discuss the ethical issue of applying "chemical restraints" in the form of sedating antipsychotic drugs.

7. Discuss review and application exercises 7, 9, and 11 (text., p. 125).

8. Use the Critical Thinking Case Study (SG, p. 35) to stimulate discussion.

Clinical Laboratory
1. For a client receiving an antipsychotic drug, ask a student to assess for sedation, hypotension, anticholinergic effects, and extrapyramidal effects, and verbally report assessment data to the instructor.

2. For a client with a nursing diagnosis of Impaired Physical Mobility related to sedation, ask the clinical group to list nursing interventions to increase client safety and decrease risks of injury.

3. For a client who has taken a phenothiazine or related antipsychotic drug for several years, have a student use the Abnormal Involuntary Movement Scale (AIMS) to assess for tardive dyskinesia.

4. For a client receiving clozapine, risperidone, or olanzapine, discuss appearances or behaviors that may indicate adverse drug reactions.

5. For a client receiving clozapine, check lab reports for decreased WBCs. If available, compare WBC values over several weeks or months. Discuss clinical manifestations and potential consequences of agranulocytosis.

TESTBANK QUESTIONS
1. Psychosis is characterized by:
    *a. disorganized and often bizarre thinking.
    b. slowed reaction time and poor coordination.
    c. manic and depressive episodes.
    d. memory deficits and dependence on others for activities of daily living.

2. All of the following drugs can cause psychosis *except:*
    a. adrenergic agents.
    b. antidepressants.
    c. anticonvulsants.
    *d. antidysrhythmics.

3. An adverse effect of phenothiazines is a decrease in:
   a. heart rate.
   b. respiratory rate.
   *c. body temperature.
   d. blood glucose.

4. Clozapine (Clozaril) produces a therapeutic effect by blocking the following receptors:
   a. Acetylcholine and glycine
   b. Epinephrine and norepinephrine
   *c. Dopamine and serotonin
   d. Aspartate and glutamate

5. A client is admitted with disruptive behavior and delusional ideations. It is important for you to do the following:
   a. Wait until the client has calmed down before doing an assessment.
   *b. Document symptoms that the client is exhibiting.
   c. Physically restrain the client.
   d. Ask the client how she feels about drug therapy.

6. A client with acute agitation, recently admitted to a psychiatric facility, is to receive a loading dose of chlorpromazine (Thorazine). The usual range for a loading dose is:
   a. 20–80 mg/day.
   b. 50–100 mg/day.
   c. 60–400 mg/day.
   *d. 400–1500 mg/day.

7. An expected outcome after 2 days of antipsychotic medication would be:
   a. absence of delusions.
   *b. increased socialization.
   c. a return to the level of functioning prior to developing psychosis.
   d. an increase in short-term memory.

8. The usual method of administering thiothixene (Navane) is by:
   a. suppository.
   b. intravenous infusion.
   c. sublingual tablet.
   *d. intramuscular injection.

9. The following statement indicates that your client has understood the teaching that you have done regarding antipsychotic medications:
   a. "I will be able to discontinue the medication if I feel better."
   b. "If I experience drowsiness I will hold the medication and call my doctor."
   *c. "Symptoms of psychosis can recur if I do not adhere to the medication schedule."
   d. "These medications are highly addictive and I must be withdrawn slowly."

10. Your client, who has been on antipsychotic medication for 2 months, begins to exhibit smacking of his lips, tongue protrusion, and facial grimacing. You will contact his physician because you suspect that he is experiencing:
    a. antiadrenergic effects of the medication.
    *b. tardive dyskinesia.
    c. anticholinergic effects of the medication.
    d. parkinsonism.

11. For clients receiving neuroleptic drugs, the following symptom should be reported immediately because it may indicate agranulocytosis:
    a. Fever
    b. Mild rash
    *c. Sore throat
    d. Diaphoresis

CRITICAL THINKING CASE STUDY

1. Antipsychotic medications are contraindicated for persons with liver damage, coronary artery disease, cerebral vascular disease, parkinsonism, bone marrow depression, severe hypotension or hypertension, coma, or severely depressed states.

2. His symptoms could be that of acute psychosis. Administer an intramuscular injection of 1.25 mg initially, then gradually increase the dose to 2.5 to 10 mg daily given in 3 to 4 divided doses.

3. Prolixin acts within hours to decrease manifestations of hyperarousal. It can be administered in various forms, including an elixir which can be mixed with a variety of noncaffeinated beverages.

4. It may take several weeks or months of drug therapy and counseling to eliminate thought disorders and increase socialization.

5. An adverse effect associated with the use of Prolixin is transient, mild drowsiness initially. The drowsiness should improve. His dosage can be adjusted if this remains a problem.

6. I will have the physician evaluate your father. There are a variety of things that this could be related to.

7. The following areas should be addressed prior to discharge: Regular blood work should be drawn to evaluate creatinine, BUN, and WBC; encourage fluids to avoid dehydration; assess for tardive dyskinesias; and tell client "do not discontinue medication if there are problems, instead contact your physician."

10
Antidepressants

MAJOR TOPICS
Unipolar and bipolar depression
Types of antidepressant drugs
Neurotransmission systems in major depression

DRUG LIST
Amitriptyline (Elavil)
Fluoxetine (Prozac)
Lithium (Eskalith, others)
Mirtazapine (Remeron)
Paroxetine (Paxil)
Sertraline (Zoloft)
Venlafaxine (Effexor)

OBJECTIVES
1. Define types and characteristics of depression.
2. Differentiate between mental depression and general CNS depression.
3. Discuss characteristics of antidepressants in terms of mechanism of action, indications for use, adverse effects, principles of therapy, and nursing process implications.
4. Compare and contrast selective serotonin reuptake inhibitors (SSRIs) with tricyclic antidepressants (TCAs).
5. List limitations for use of monoamine oxidase (MAO) inhibitor antidepressants.
6. Describe the use of lithium in bipolar disorder.
7. Discuss interventions to increase safety of lithium therapy.
8. Describe the nursing role in preventing, recognizing, and treating overdoses of antidepressant drugs and lithium.

TEACHING STRATEGIES

Classroom

1. Ask students what appearances and behaviors would make them think a client is depressed.
2. Ask students about ways to distinguish between temporary sadness that does not require drug therapy and major depression that often does require drug therapy.
3. Show a transparency of the major groups of antidepressants (IM, p. 136).
4. Discuss TCAs as the prototypes and SSRIs as the most commonly used drugs.
5. Compare TCAs and SSRIs in terms of adverse drug effects.
6. Have students write brief descriptions of the mechanism of action for major types of antidepressants.
7. Discuss the importance of teaching clients that optimal therapeutic effects may not occur until they have been taking the drug for 2 to 3 weeks.

8. Discuss laboratory monitoring of clients taking lithium.
9. Discuss the rationale for adequate sodium intake during lithium therapy.
10. Assign the Critical Thinking Case Study (SG, p. 38) as homework, then discuss as a class.

Clinical Laboratory

1. With a client receiving an SSRI antidepressant drug, ask a student to interview the client regarding therapeutic and adverse effects. Results may be discussed in a postconference or written and turned in to the instructor.
2. For a client with a nursing diagnosis of Knowledge Deficit related to effects and appropriate usage of antidepressant drugs, have a student prepare a teaching plan.
3. Discuss ways to assist clients in maintaining usual activities of daily living, when feasible, while taking an antidepressant drug as an outpatient.
4. On a hospital unit with medical-surgical patients, assign one or more students to review medication administration records and list the patients receiving an antidepressant. This exercise can increase students' awareness of depression as a symptom in nonpsychiatric illnesses.
5. In home care of a depressed client, have a student assess the risk of suicide, the ability and willingness to take antidepressant medication as prescribed, the use of other drugs that stimulate or depress CNS function, and the availability of social support systems. Have the student intervene to promote compliance, safety, and well-being when indicated.

TESTBANK QUESTIONS

1. The following assertion by Mr. Z. leads you to believe that he understands the teaching you have done regarding amitriptyline (Elavil). He will take the medication:
   a. for 2 to 3 weeks.
   b. until his symptoms subside.
   *c. for several months.
   d. for the rest of his life.
2. A client is admitted to your unit because of an overdose of doxepin (Sinequan). Which of the following nursing diagnoses would be a priority?
   a. Risk for injury related to sedation
   b. Knowledge deficit related to effects and usage of antidepressants
   c. Nutritional disturbances related to nausea, anorexia, and weight loss
   *d. Decreased cardiac output related to hypotension

3. Which of the following statements by your client, who is being discharged on a TCA, would lead you to believe that he needs additional discharge instructions?
   *a. "I can drink 1 beer daily and it will not cause any problems."
   b. "I must stop smoking cigarettes."
   c. "I will check with the pharmacist before I buy any over-the-counter medications."
   d. "I will tell my dentist before he gives me any medications that I am taking an antidepressant."

4. Mr. S. is started on amitriptyline (Elavil), a tricyclic antidepressant. Which information should be included in Mr. S.'s teaching plan? "You should:
   *a. sit on the side of your bed before getting up and stand up very slowly."
   b. increase foods that are high in potassium in your diet."
   c. elevate your legs whenever you sit down."
   d. eat six small meals throughout the day."

5. A deficiency of the following electrolyte will predispose a client who is using lithium to toxicity:
   *a. Sodium
   b. Potassium
   c. Chloride
   d. Magnesium

6. Which of the following medications, if administered concurrently with lithium, could produce a toxic effect?
   a. Prednisone
   b. Digoxin (Lanoxin)
   c. Insulin
   *d. Furosemide (Lasix)

7. J. was admitted with agitation and hyperactivity related to bipolar affective disorder. After 5 days of treatment with lithium, he complains of feeling slowed down and has increased thirst but remains hyperactive. Your analysis is that:
   a. your client remains manic but has developed toxic side effects from lithium.
   *b. your client remains manic without serious side effects of toxicity.
   c. the treatment has been ineffective; he should be calm at this time.
   d. a higher dose is required to achieve a therapeutic effect.

8. Foods that should be avoided when a person is taking phenelzine (Nardil) include:
   a. citrus fruits.
   b. dark green vegetables.
   *c. aged cheeses.
   d. red meat.

9. Your client is to be started on phenelzine (Nardil), an MAO inhibitor. The following should be monitored frequently:
   *a. Blood pressure
   b. Lung sounds
   c. Serum creatinine
   d. Hemoglobin

10. You are giving instructions prior to your client being discharged on tranyl-cypromine (Parnate). You know your teaching has been effective if he states that concurrent use of foods high in tyramine can cause:
    a. nausea, anorexia, and weight loss.
    b. orthostatic hypotension.
    *c. hypertensive crisis.
    d. hallucinations.

11. Your client is started on an MAO inhibitor for depression. He should avoid:
    a. caffeine.
    b. eggs.
    c. red meat.
    *d. red wine.

12. Clients who are receiving bupropion (Wellbutrin) are at increased risk for developing:
    a. acne.
    *b. seizures.
    c. coronary artery disease.
    d. diabetes mellitus.

13. Your client asks you when he can expect to see a therapeutic response from fluoxetine (Prozac), the best response would be:
    a. 24–48 hours.
    b. 7–10 days.
    *c. 2–3 weeks.
    d. 6–8 weeks.

14. Which of the following statements by Mrs. G. would lead you to believe that she has a good understanding of the adverse effects of fluoxetine (Prozac)?
    a. "I will need additional sleep while I am taking this medication."
    *b. "If I develop a rash, I will contact my physician."
    c. "It will take 4 weeks before I feel a therapeutic effect from this medication."
    d. "I must increase my fluid intake while I am taking this medication."

CRITICAL THINKING CASE STUDY

1. A client admitted with depression is assessed for the following symptoms: loss of energy, fatigue, indecisiveness, difficulty thinking and concentrating, loss of interest in appearance, feelings of worthlessness, change in weight or appetite, sleep disorders, and obsession with death. If the client has 5 of these symptoms, it would constitute a major depression.

2. The two illnesses that should be considered prior to prescribing medication are diabetes mellitus and chronic lung disease. TCAs and lithium can cause weight gain which could affect diabetic control. If the individual with chronic lung disease is still smoking, that can decrease the effect of the TCAs. A diabetic taking MAO inhibitors can experience hypoglycemia. Persons with chronic lung disease can have dyspnea as a result of SSRIs.

3. The client will experience improvement of mood. The client will resume self-care activities.

4. Teach the client and caretaker: to take antidepressive drugs as directed, that the therapeutic effects may not occur for 2 to 3 weeks, not to take other drugs without contacting their physician, to tell other health care providers that they are taking this medication.

5. Observe for behaviors indicating lessening of depresson and observe for suicide thoughts and behaviors. Also evaluate the client for weight loss.

6. Speak with the physicians about the client's unwillingness.

11
Anticonvulsants

MAJOR TOPICS
Causes and types of seizure disorders
Treatment of seizure disorders

DRUG LIST
Carbamazepine (Tegretol)
Clonazepam (Klonopin)
Fosphenytoin (Cerebyx)
Gabapentin (Neurontin)
Lamotrigine (Lamictal)
Phenytoin (Dilantin)
Valproic acid (Depakene, Depakote)

OBJECTIVES
1. Define terms commonly used to describe seizure disorders.
2. Discuss major factors that influence the choice of an anticonvulsant drug for a client with a seizure disorder.
3. Differentiate uses and effects of commonly used anticonvulsant drugs.
4. Apply the nursing process with clients experiencing selected seizure disorders.

TEACHING STRATEGIES

Classroom
1. Lecture/discussion regarding selected anticonvulsant drugs. Of the listed drugs, carbamazepine, clonazepam, phenytoin, and valproic acid are in the top 200 outpatient drugs.
2. Discuss advantages and disadvantages of the various drugs in terms of efficacy and adverse effects.
3. Discuss the rationale for using a single drug when possible (monotherapy versus polytherapy).
4. Discuss dosage and administration of fosphenytoin.
5. Discuss the importance of teaching clients on long-term anticonvulsant therapy not to stop taking their medication abruptly or without their physician's consent and supervision.
6. Describe the nursing care needed by a client experiencing an acute tonic-clonic convulsion.
7. Use the Critical Thinking Case Study (SG, p. 23) as a basis for class discussion.

Clinical Laboratory
1. Ask students to identify clients at risk of having acute seizure or status epilepticus.
2. For clients receiving an anticonvulsant drug, have students assess perceptions of the disease process, the prescribed drug therapy, and compliance with the prescribed treatment regimen.
3. For clients receiving an anticonvulsant drug, have students verbalize at least one drug therapy related nursing diagnosis to the instructor.
4. For clients known to have epilepsy, have students assess the ability of family members or caregivers to recognize and appropriately manage an acute seizure.
5. Determine the agency's procedure for rapidly obtaining IV diazepam or lorazepam when a patient has a convulsion or status epilepticus. In postconference, discuss the procedure and have students role play the nursing process for a patient experiencing a tonic-clonic seizure.

TESTBANK QUESTIONS
1. Carbamazepine (Tegretol) may also be used for the treatment of:
   a. Parkinson's disease.
   *b. trigeminal neuralgia.
   c. Bell's palsy.
   d. hiccups.

2. Mr. J. is admitted with acute alcohol intoxication. Which medication should you administer to prevent Mr. J. from experiencing seizures as he undergoes alcohol withdrawal?
   a. Primidone (Mysoline)
   b. Ethosuximide (Zarontin)
   *c. Clorazepate (Tranxene)
   d. Phenytoin (Dilantin)

3. Mr. J.'S Dilantin level is 25 µg/ml. Based on this level you would:
   a. continue the dose as ordered.
   b. decrease the daily dose.
   *c. hold the drug until further orders.
   d. increase the daily dose.

4. J.K. is experiencing continuous seizures. Which of the following medications is the most effective in treating status epilepticus?
   a. Clonazepam (Klonopin)
   b. Carbamazepine (Tegretol)
   c. Ethosuximide (Zarontin)
   *d. Diazepam (Valium)

5. R.F. is to be sent home on Dilantin 100 mg b.i.d. Which of the following statements by R.F. lead you to believe that he has understood your teaching?
   a. "I will take the medication on an empty stomach."
   b. "I will discontinue the drug immediately if any side effects occur."
   *c. "I will make routine visits to the dentist."
   d. "I will weigh myself daily."

6. An adverse effect of the administration of phenobarbital is:
   *a. anemia.
   b. bradycardia.
   c. cravings.
   d. double vision.

7. You are writing a nursing outcome for J.R. who has partial seizures. Which of the following would be appropriate? J.R. will experience:
   *a. control of partial seizures.
   b. absence of drug side effects.
   c. seizure control without medications.
   d. no further seizure activity.

8. For clients receiving carbamazepine (Tegretol), the following electrolyte value should be monitored:
   a. Zinc
   b. Potassium
   *c. Calcium
   d. Chloride

9. Mrs. C., who has had a seizure disorder since childhood that is controlled by anticonvulsant medication, asks you if she should become pregnant. Identify the best response:
   a. "Since you have been on the medication for such a long time, your chances of having a healthy pregnancy are good."
   *b. "There is an increased risk of birth defects in women who are taking anticonvulsants during their pregnancy."
   c. "You should avoid becoming pregnant because your chances of carrying the baby to term are slim."
   d. "If you watch your diet very closely, the doctor may be able to take you off of your medication so that you can become pregnant."

10. Which of the following adverse effects of Dilantin would necessitate that it be discontinued?
    a. Hiccups
    b. Blurred vision
    *c. Rash
    d. Dry cough

11. J.K. is started on valproic acid (Depakene). Which of the following lab studies should be monitored regularly?
    *a. SGOT/AST and LDH
    b. Creatinine and BUN
    c. PT and PTT
    d. Serum sodium and potassium levels

12. When lorazepam (Ativan) is being administered intravenously for the rapid control of tonic-clonic seizures, the nurse needs to observe the client for:
    a. hemorrhage.
    b. dysrhythmias.
    *c. respiratory depression.
    d. hypertension.

13. When phenobarbital is being administered with other medications, the dosage of the other drug(s) may need to be adjusted because phenobarbital:
    *a. can accelerate the rate of drug metabolism.
    b. inhibits liver enzyme formation.
    c. can potentiate hepatotoxicity.
    d. inhibits excretion of drug metabolites.

14. Which of the common adverse effects associated with anticonvulsant therapy can be avoided with effective teaching?
    a. Diplopia
    b. Urticaria
    *c. Nausea
    d. Ataxia

15. Miss T., a 38-year-old insulin-dependent diabetic, has just been brought to the emergency room because of a seizure. Miss T. has no history of a seizure disorder. A possible cause for the seizure is:
    *a. hypoglycemia.
    b. hyponatremia.
    c. acidosis.
    d. anaphylactic reaction.

16. The drug of choice for treating generalized seizures in children under the age of 2 months is:
    a. ethosuximide (Zarontin).
    b. clonazepam (Klonopin).
    c. phenytoin (Dilantin).
    *d. phenobarbital.

17. If the intravenous line is not flushed prior to administering phenytoin (Dilantin) intravenously, the following will occur:
    a. The client's blood pressure will drop.
    *b. The solution will crystallize in the line.
    c. The client's heart will fibrillate.
    d. The line will turn amber.

18. Administration of anticonvulsants for long periods can cause decreased folic acid levels, which results in:
    a. iron deficiency anemia.
    b. pellagra.
    c. pernicious anemia.
    *d. megaloblastic anemia.

19. The dosage of phenytoin (Dilantin) may need to be increased if your client is taking:
    a. cimetidine (Tagamet).
    b. diazepam (Valium).
    c. amitriptyline (Elavil).
    *d. theophylline (Theo-Dur).

20. This drug may be used alone or with other anticonvulsants to treat myoclonic or akinetic seizures:
    a. Ethosuximide (Zarontin)
    *b. Clonazepam (Klonopin)
    c. Phenytoin (Dilantin)
    d. Diazepam (Valium)

21. Abrupt withdrawal of clonazepam (Klonopin) may result in:
    a. increased intracranial pressure.
    b. hyperactivity.
    *c. status epilepticus.
    d. migraine headaches.

CRITICAL THINKING CASE STUDY

1. Stay with her and prevent her from hurting herself. Make sure that she can breathe adequately; time and observe the characteristics of the seizure.

2. The larger the anticonvulsant dose, the greater the possibility of adverse effects. Therefore, it is better to use two anticonvulsants at lower doses to control seizures.

3. Contact her physician immediately. One or both of the medications may need to be discontinued.

4. There is no way of knowing at this time how long C.M. may need to be on the medications. It is common practice to keep the person on medication for a year post-injury or until the person has been seizure free for a year. There is a possi-

bility that C.M. may need to be on the medication the rest of her life depending upon the extent of her injury.

5. Therapeutic serum levels take about 2–3 weeks, and a steady-state concentration takes 3–4 weeks. Take the drug exactly as the doctor prescribes, it must not be stopped abruptly. Report any seizure activity to the doctor, including excessive drowsiness, in which case the doctor may be able to adjust the dosage. Carry identification that contains the medical information that would be needed in the event the seizure took place in public or there was an emergency situation. See the dentist regularly. Take the medications with food to prevent GI upsets.

12
Antiparkinson Drugs

MAJOR TOPICS

Idiopathic Parkinson's disease
Types of antiparkinson drugs

DRUG LIST

Benztropine (Cogentin)
Levodopa/carbidopa (Sinemet)
Selegiline (Eldepryl)
Trihexyphenidyl (Artane)

OBJECTIVES

1. Describe major characteristics of Parkinson's disease.
2. Differentiate the types of commonly used antiparkinson drugs.
3. Discuss therapeutic and adverse effects of dopaminergic and anticholinergic drugs.
4. Apply nursing process with clients experiencing parkinsonism.

TEACHING STRATEGIES

Classroom

1. Discuss the dopaminergic and anticholinergic effects of antiparkinson drugs.

2. Contrast treatment of idiopathic and drug-induced parkinsonism.

3. Assign or discuss the Critical Thinking Case study (SG, p. 45).

Clinical Laboratory

1. For a client known to have Parkinson's disease, have a student assess for therapeutic and adverse effects of prescribed drugs.

2. For a client receiving older antipsychotic drugs, have a student assess for signs and symptoms of parkinsonism.

TESTBANK QUESTIONS

1. Mr. C. is presently taking trihexyphenidyl (Artane), and his physician has now added Sinemet. Which of the following statements by Mr. C. leads you to believe that he has understood your teaching regarding this medication?
   a. "This drug will eliminate all of my symptoms."
   *b. "Long-term use of this drug may cause movement disturbances."
   c. "I will take this drug with a high-protein meal."
   d. "I will need to take a high-potency vitamin containing vitamin K."

2. Pseudoparkinsonism may occur with long-term use of:
   *a. antipsychotics.
   b. psychedelics.
   c. antidepressants.
   d. sedative-hypnotics.

3. When teaching your client about trihexyphenidyl (Artane), it is important to instruct her that because of the additive anticholinergic effect she needs to avoid the concurrent use of:
   a. aspirin compounds.
   *b. antihistamines.
   c. alcohol.
   d. aminoglycosides.

4. Which of the following statements by your client indicates a lack of understanding of Parkinson's disease?
   a. "Tremors are aggravated by stress and tend to disappear during sleep."
   b. "Intelligence is not impaired in most people with Parkinson's."
   *c. "Advanced parkinsonism is more likely to respond to levodopa than earlier stages of the disease.
   d. "Decrease in dopamine activity is responsible for the development of Parkinson's disease."

5. Carbidopa is frequently used with levodopa because it:
   a. increases metabolism of levodopa.
   *b. results in less levodopa being decarboxylated in the periphery.
   c. increases the production of dopamine in the brain.
   d. inhibits reuptake of dopamine in the brain.

6. Which of the following statements by Mrs. G. leads you to believe that she does not understand the teaching that you have done regarding levodopa?
   a. "Persons taking levodopa should not take diuretics concurrently."
   *b. "If I become nauseated, I will withhold the medication."
   c. "I can still have an occasional glass of wine."
   d. "I will increase my vitamin C intake."

7. Mrs. P., a 76-year-old retired nurse, is taking amantadine hydrochloride (Symmetrel). Which of the following statements by Mrs. P. leads you to believe that she needs additional teaching?
   a. "This drug is also used to treat viral infections."
   b. "This drug can accumulate in persons with decreased renal function."
   c. "Tremor and rigidity will improve within a few weeks after I begin to take this medication."
   *d. "This drug can decrease mental alertness."

8. Which of the following vitamins is an antagonist to levodopa?
   a. B1 (thiamine)
   *b. B6 (pyridoxine)
   c. B2 (riboflavin)
   d. C (ascorbic acid)

9. When trihexyphenidyl (Artane) and Sinemet are administered concurrently, there is a potential for altered absorption of Sinemet due to the effect of trihexyphenidyl, which
   a. reduces lipid solubility.
   b. enhances first-pass effect.
   c. increases gastric motility.
   *d. delays gastric emptying.

10. Which of the following should the nurse be assessing for when Sinemet is administered?
    *a. Irregular heart rate
    b. Elevated blood pressure
    c. Decreased urinary output
    d. Gingival hyperplasia

11. Clients receiving anticholinergic agents for Parkinson's disease should be aware that a common adverse effect of the medication is:
    a. blood dyscrasias.
    b. dizziness.
    *c. dry mouth.
    d. diarrhea.

12. Your client is being treated for diabetes mellitus. Her physician has recently diagnosed her with Parkinson's disease. For which of the following would an anticholinergic agent be contraindicated?
    a. Diverticulitis
    b. Diabetes mellitus
    *c. Glaucoma
    d. Hypertension

13. Concurrent administration of an anticholinergic, antiparkinson agent with a phenothiazine agent can cause:
    *a. paralytic ileus and hypothermia.
    b. vomiting and epigastric distress.
    c. blurred vision and vertigo.
    d. confusion and disorientation.

14. The administration of benztropine (Cogentin) is contraindicated in the presence of:
    a. diabetes mellitus.
    *b. tardive dyskinesia.
    c. renal insufficiency.
    d. pulmonary fibrosis.

15. You know that your teaching has been effective when a client with Parkinson's disease on levodopa (Larodopa) states, "I will:
    a. increase the dose when the tremors or stiffness become worse."
    *b. take the medication with milk or at mealtime to decrease stomach irritation."
    c. include a multivitamin in my daily routine for balanced nutrition."
    d. notify my physician if my urine or perspiration turns a darker color."

16. Before giving medication to a client with Parkinson's disease, you must first assess all of the following *except:*
    a. medication allergies.
    b. other medical problems.
    *c. family support.
    d. condition of his skin.

17. Your client recently started taking levodopa. The following dietary change should be stressed:
    a. Avoid rich, fatty foods.
    *b. Limit foods high in protein.
    c. Eat small frequent meals.
    d. Avoid foods high in sodium.

18. Your client on levodopa states, "Just take all those pills away; they are not doing me any good." The nurse's best response would be:
    *a. "You believe that the pills are not helping."
    b. "It sounds to me like you are angry."
    c. "Where did you get the idea that the pills are not helping?"
    d. "Does it upset you to have to take medication?"

CRITICAL THINKING CASE STUDY

1. Anticholinergic agents are commonly the drugs of choice when symptoms are relatively mild.

2. Adverse effects of the medication and nursing interventions:
   a. Tachycardia and palpitations are usually not serious; contact physician if problematic.
   b. For tremors and restlessness, contact physician to adjust dose.
   c. For sedation and drowsiness, if excessive, adjust dose.
   d. For constipation, treat with fluids, roughage, exercise, and laxatives.

3. Parkinson's disease progresses at different rates in individuals. The symptoms can be controlled with medications.

4. Levodopa and carbidopa are the drugs of choice when bradykinesia and rigidity are the predominant symptoms.

5. Excessive dryness of mouth can be minimized with adequate hydration. Alcohol and high protein foods should be limited. Do not take vitamins containing B_6, because B_6 can decrease the effects of antiparkinson medications. Report any adverse effects.

13
Skeletal Muscle Relaxants

MAJOR TOPICS

Musculoskeletal pain and spasm
Multiple sclerosis

DRUG LIST

Baclofen (Lioresal)
Carisoprodol (Rela, Soma)
Cyclobenzaprine (Flexeril)
Dantrolene (Dantrium)
Diazepam (Valium)

OBJECTIVES

1. Discuss common symptoms/disorders for which skeletal muscle relaxants are used.
2. Differentiate uses and effects of selected drugs.
3. Describe nonpharmacologic interventions to relieve muscle spasm and spasticity.
4. Apply nursing process with clients experiencing muscle spasm and spasticity.

TEACHING STRATEGIES

Classroom

1. Discuss acute musculoskeletal injury (e.g., ankle sprain) and multiple sclerosis as conditions in which these drugs are used.

2. Discuss nonpharmacologic treatments of muscle spasm, musculoskeletal pain, and spasticity.

3. Differentiate between centrally active and peripherally active drugs.

4. Discuss the Critical Thinking Case Study (SG, p. 49).

Clinical Laboratory

1. For a client with a nursing diagnosis of Self-Care Deficit related to spasm and pain, list the interventions needed.

2. For a client with multiple sclerosis, assess comfort level and functional ability in usual activities of daily living.

3. Interview a client with multiple sclerosis regarding his or her perceptions of "helping behaviors" from nurses and other health-care providers.

TESTBANK QUESTIONS

1. A common adverse reaction seen in individuals taking centrally acting muscle relaxants is:
   a. muscle spasms.
   *b. ataxia.
   c. insomnia.
   d. excessive salivation.

2. The following muscle relaxant, administered intravenously, is used to manage intraoperative hyperthermia:
   a. Carisoprodol (Soma)
   *b. Dantrolene (Dantrium)
   c. Baclofen (Lioresal)
   d. Methocarbamol (Robaxin)

3. The disorder that may be aggravated by the administration of muscle relaxants is:
   a. angina.
   b. peripheral edema.
   c. esophageal reflux.
   *d. tachycardia.

4. The most effective muscle relaxant for treating problems associated with multiple sclerosis is:
   a. methocarbamol (Robaxin).
   b. diazepam (Valium).
   *c. baclofen (Lioresal).
   d. orphenadrine citrate (Norflex).

5. Muscle spasms can be decreased by muscle relaxants and the concurrent use of:
   a. anti-inflammatory drugs.
   *b. moist heat.
   c. steroids.
   d. passive range of motion.

6. Administered intravenously, this drug is used to treat muscle spasms:
   a. Metaxalone (Skelaxin)
   b. Carisoprodol (Rela, Soma)
   c. Baclofen (Lioresal)
   *d. Diazepam (Valium)

7. The following lab studies should be assessed before dantrolene (Dantrium) is administered:
   a. Serum glucose
   b. Serum potassium
   c. Lipase and amylase
   *d. SGOT and LDH

8. Which of the following statements by a 76-year-old client leads you to believe that he understood your teaching regarding baclofen (Lioresal)?
   a. "I will take my medication on an empty stomach."
   b. "I will increase my intake of foods high in vitamin C."
   *c. "I will contact my physician if I experience vomiting and diarrhea.
   d. "Skin rashes are expected and will go away in a few weeks."

CRITICAL THINKING CASE STUDY

1. Assess his mobility and pain level. Look for any swelling or tenderness. Ask him if he has been following the doctor's directions.

2. This medication is for short-term use. The maximum recommended duration is 3 weeks.

3. Other therapies include moist heat, massage, exercise, and relaxation techniques.

14
Anesthetics

MAJOR TOPICS

Types of anesthesia
General and local anesthetics
Perioperative adjunctive drugs
Nurse's role in preoperative and postoperative care

OBJECTIVES

1. Discuss factors considered when choosing an anesthetic agent.
2. Describe characteristics of general and regional anesthetic agents.
3. Compare general and local anesthetics in terms of administration, client safety, and nursing care.
4. Discuss the rationale for using adjunctive drugs before and during surgical procedures.
5. Describe the nurse's role in relation to anesthetics and adjunctive drugs.

TEACHING STRATEGIES

Classroom

1. Lecture/discussion of types and characteristics of general and regional anesthesia.
2. Ask students for personal experiences or their observations of clients before and after surgery.
3. Describe the appearance and care of a client in the immediate postoperative period following general inhalational anesthesia.
4. Discuss the Critical Thinking Case Study (SG, p. 52).

Clinical Laboratory

1. For a postoperative client, have a student review operative records, list preoperative medications, list anesthetic and other intraoperative drugs, and discuss implications for postoperative nursing care.
2. In an ambulatory surgery center or emergency room, have a student observe or assist with a minor procedure requiring local anesthesia.

TESTBANK QUESTIONS

1. The following is a manifestation of stage I anesthesia:
   *a. Excitement and hyperactivity
   b. Rapid loss of consciousness
   c. Medullary paralysis
   d. No spontaneous breathing

2. An adverse effect of halothane (Fluothane) is:
   a. increased risk of laryngospasm.
   b. severe nausea and vomiting.
   c. increased tracheobronchial secretions.
   *d. cardiac dysrhythmias.

3. A contraindication for the use of methoxyflurane (Penthrane) is:
   a. heart failure.
   *b. renal impairment.
   c. glaucoma.
   d. diabetes mellitus.

4. Etomidate (Amidate) is best used for:
   a. induction of anesthesia.
   b. diagnostic procedures.
   *c. short-term operative procedures.
   d. major surgical procedures.

5. Inhalation anesthetics are removed from the body by the:
   a. kidneys.
   b. liver.
   c. intestines.
   *d. lungs.

6. Narcotic analgesics are given preoperatively:
   a. to minimize the amount of analgesic needed postoperatively.
   b. to induce anesthesia.
   *c. to induce relaxation.
   d. so that the induction process will be more rapid.

7. Nursing measures appropriate for all clients in the recovery room after anesthesia include:
   a. assessing for a gag reflex.
   b. providing passive range of motion.
   c. assessing output hourly.
   *d. monitoring respiratory status.

8. The most commonly used local anesthetic is:
   a. procaine (Novocaine).
   *b. lidocaine (Xylocaine).
   c. tetracaine (Pontocaine).
   d. mepivacaine (Carbocaine).

9. A drug used for topical anesthesia of the nose and ear is:
   a. benzocaine (Americaine).
   b. bupivacaine (Marcaine).
   *c. cocaine.
   d. etidocaine (Duranest).

10. Anticholinergic drugs are used preoperatively to prevent:
    a. hypertension postoperatively.
    b. urination during surgery.
    c. peristalsis.
    *d. excessive parasympathetic nervous system activity.

CRITICAL THINKING CASE STUDY

1. Other situations in which this type of anesthesia may be used includes perineal and rectal surgery.

2. The duration of the block can vary depending on the type of block and the drug concentration. When you feel an urge to void, call the nurse so she can assist you because hypotension can occur after spinal anesthesia.

3. What Mrs. J. will be able to feel will depend upon the site of injection and the level to which the drug rises in the spinal column. It will be a number of hours before Mrs. J. will have full mobility and sensation in her lower extremities.

4. The fetal responses to anesthesia may include depressed muscle strength, muscle tone, and rooting behavior.

5. The infant should be assessed regularly after delivery. The depressed rooting behavior may make breast feeding more challenging initially and the mother should be reassured that this is temporary.

6. Urinary retention is common after spinal surgery. The nurse should assess Mrs. J. for bladder distention. If she has been NPO for a number of hours she may not need to void at this time. If her bladder is distended and she is uncomfortable, you should contact the physician.

15
Alcohol and Other Drug Abuse

MAJOR TOPICS

Drug abuse and dependence
Physiologic effects of alcohol, cocaine, and marijuana
Withdrawal reactions
Treatment of abuse and dependence

DRUG LIST

Cocaine
Disulfiram (Antabuse)
Ethanol
Heroin
Levo-alpha-acetylmethadol (LAAM) (Orlaam)
Marijuana
Naltrexone (Trexan)
Nicotine (Nicoderm, Nicorette)

OBJECTIVES

1. Identify risk factors for developing drug dependence.
2. Describe the effects of alcohol, cocaine, and marijuana on selected body organs.
3. Compare and contrast characteristics of dependence associated with alcohol, benzodiazepines, cocaine, and opiates.
4. Describe specific antidotes for overdoses of CNS depressant drugs and the circumstances indicating their use.
5. Outline major elements of treatment for overdoses of commonly abused drugs that do not have antidotes.
6. Describe interventions to prevent or manage withdrawal reactions associated with benzodiazepines, cocaine and other CNS stimulants, ethanol, and opiates.
7. Assign or discuss the Critical Thinking Case Study (SG, p. 56).

TEACHING STRATEGIES

Classroom

1. Discuss assessment of clients in relation to risks of abusing drugs.
2. Discuss management of clients with acute or chronic alcohol intoxication.
3. Discuss the rationale for administering sedatives to clients with alcohol dependence.
4. Review administration of flumazenil and naloxone.
5. Discuss nurses as a high-risk group for abusing drugs.
6. Discuss ethical and legal implications of nurses who divert clients' drugs to themselves.
7. Discuss the use of LAAM or methadone in treatment of heroin addiction.
8. Discuss the use of nicotine replacement in smoking cessation regimens.

Clinical Laboratory

1. For a client receiving benzodiazepines or opiates, assign a student to assess for manifestations of abuse, dependence, and overdose.
2. For a client who acts intoxicated during hospitalization, review medical records and interview visitors to assess prehospitalization behavior and possible causes of the behavior.
3. In organized health care settings, review agency policies about the handling of psychotropic and narcotic drugs.
4. In home care settings, assess all members of the household in relation to possible alcohol or other drug abuse.

TESTBANK QUESTIONS

1. An 18-year-old male is brought into the ER because a barbiturate overdose is suspected; you should observe him for:
   *a. respiratory depression.
   b. electrolyte imbalance.
   c. impaired clotting.
   d. bone marrow depression.

2. A 10-year-old male at the school where you are a nurse has recently exhibited violent behavior, his grades have plummeted, and he has withdrawn from soccer. You suspect he may be using:
   a. amphetamines.
   b. marijuana.
   c. narcotics.
   *d. inhalants.

3. Persons using narcotics routinely will experience:
   a. anxiety.
   b. bradycardia.
   *c. constipation.
   d. diarrhea.

4. Frequent use of the following recreational drug can cause infertility:
   a. Alcohol
   b. Pentobarbital
   *c. Cannabis
   d. Darvon

5. When alcoholics are admitted to the hospital, they should be evaluated for:
   a. pulmonary edema.
   b. bone marrow depression.
   c. hypertension.
   *d. vitamin deficiencies.

6. Alcohol withdrawal is treated with chlordiazepoxide (librium) to prevent:
   a. anoxia.
   b. hypotension.
   *c. convulsions.
   d. gastrointestinal bleeding.

7. Acute psychosis can occur as a result of ingesting:
   a. alcohol.
   *b. hallucinogens.
   c. barbiturates.
   d. narcotics.

8. Which of the following substances produces an intense psychological dependence from initial trial?
   a. Amphetamines
   b. Barbiturates
   *c. Cocaine
   d. Dilaudid

9. The following recreational drug may cause hallucinations and "flashbacks":
   a. Cocaine
   b. Methadone
   c. Heroin
   *d. LSD

10. Your 16-year-old daughter tells you that she has started smoking to temporarily help control her weight. Considering the developmental age of the child, what *best* response would dissuade her from smoking?
    *a. It will also stain your teeth, give you foul smelling breath, and predispose you to wrinkles.
    b. It will also greatly increase your risk of developing emphysema in later life.
    c. Of course you know that you are placing yourself at risk for many different types of cancer.
    d. It is very difficult to smoke for a short period of time because cigarettes are habit forming.

11. Which of the following statements leads you to believe that the individual understands the dangers of using substances of abuse?
    a. "Herbal stimulants cannot cause you any harm because they are sold at health food stores."
    *b. "Barbiturates can result in liver damage."
    c. "Persons using marijuana on a regular basis have not demonstrated any adverse physical effects."
    d. "I will not take narcotics after surgery because I can become addicted."

12. When administering drugs to alcoholic patients taking disulfiram (Antabuse), the nurse should avoid:
    *a. elixirs.
    b. magmas.
    c. syrups.
    d. lozenges.

CRITICAL THINKING CASE STUDY

1. The nurse needs to identify health problems, allergies, medications, and social habits, including daily alcohol and drug intake. The nurse should also find out if M. is being followed by a physician.

2. Ingestion of alcohol during pregnancy can cause fetal alcohol syndrome.

3. M. is symptomatic and needs to be medicated. Normally benzodiazepines such as Librium are used to prevent delirium tremens. Any medication administered during pregnancy must be evaluated for its detrimental effects to the fetus.

4. Delirium tremens are characterized by confusion, disorientation, delusion, and hallucinations.

5. Antepartum care should be discussed, including proper nutrition. M.'s smoking also needs to be addressed because of the harmful effects to the fetus.

6. Referrals the nurse should make include: the health department/visiting nurse association, an alcoholic rehabilitation program, and a physician for follow-up.

7. If alcohol is ingested concurrently with Antabuse, flushing, dyspnea, hypotension, tachycardia, nausea, vomiting, syncope, vertigo, blurred vision, headache, confusion, respiratory depression, dysrhythmia, myocardial infarction, unconsciousness, convulsions, or death can occur. The same type of reaction can also occur when certain drugs are ingested with Antabuse.

16
Central Nervous System Stimulants

MAJOR TOPICS

Amphetamines and related drugs
Disorders for which CNS stimulants are used

DRUG LIST

Caffeine
Dextroamphetamine (Dexedrine)
Methylphenidate (Ritalin)

OBJECTIVES

1. Describe general characteristics of CNS stimulant drugs.
2. Discuss reasons for decreased use of amphetamines for therapeutic purposes.
3. Discuss the rationale for treating ADHD with CNS stimulant drugs.
4. Describe characteristics and effects of xanthine drugs.

TEACHING STRATEGIES

Classroom

1. Some authorities think ADHD is too frequently diagnosed and treated with CNS stimulants. Assign two groups of students to debate this issue.

2. Discuss potential therapeutic and adverse effects of CNS stimulant therapy in children.

Clinical Laboratory

1. In a school, outpatient clinic, or physician's office, observe a child diagnosed with ADHD and compare his or her

behavior with the behavior of a similar-aged child without ADHD.

2. Prepare a teaching plan for parents of a child who has methylphenidate newly prescribed for ADHD.

TESTBANK QUESTIONS

1. An expected outcome after the administration of methylphenidate (Ritalin) is:
   a. elimination of behavioral problems.
   *b. increased attention span.
   c. increased intellectual capacity.
   d. improvement in fine motor skills.

2. The following statement by the parents of a child receiving methylphenidate indicates that they understand how the drug is to be used.
   a. "I know that my child can develop a tolerance to the medication, so we will monitor him."
   *b. "Drug holidays will be used to evaluate his behavioral response to the medication."
   c. "Self-image and learning ability may diminish with the use of this drug."
   d. "Stimulants used for ADHD always produce a therapeutic effect."

3. Children using methylphenidate should be taught to avoid foods containing:
   a. tyramine.
   b. sodium.
   *c. caffeine.
   d. potassium.

4. Your client has started taking amphetamines for narcolepsy. He should be instructed to report the following adverse effect of the medication:
   a. Increased motor activity
   b. Anorexia
   *c. Tachycardia and palpitations
   d. Constipation

5. Caffeine:
   a. does not produce tolerance.
   b. does not cause habituation.
   *c. can be used to treat migraine headaches.
   d. should be avoided by persons with respiratory problems.

6. Doxapram (Dopram):
   *a. increases respiratory rate.
   b. decreases oxygen consumption.
   c. decreases carbon dioxide production.
   d. increases cardiac output.

III
DRUGS AFFECTING THE
AUTONOMIC NERVOUS SYSTEM

17
Physiology of the Autonomic Nervous System

MAJOR TOPICS

General characteristics and functions of the sympathetic nervous system (SNS)
General characteristics and functions of the parasympathetic nervous system (PNS)
Overview of autonomic nervous system (ANS) drugs

OBJECTIVES

1. Identify physiologic effects of the SNS.
2. Differentiate subtypes and functions of SNS receptors.
3. Identify physiologic effects of the PNS.
4. Differentiate subtypes and functions of PNS receptors.
5. State names and general characteristics of drugs affecting the ANS.

TEACHING STRATEGIES

Classroom

1. Student knowledge about the ANS, including receptors, is essential to understanding how drugs increase or decrease ANS functions. Thus, a relatively detailed review and discussion may be needed.

2. Assign or recommend reviewing the autonomic nervous system in a physiology or pathophysiology text.

3. To focus students' attention, have them count their own heart rates while seated, stand and do "jumping jack" exercises for 2–3 minutes, then count their heart rates again. Ask "What have we done in relation to today's topic?" The answer is: "We've activated our sympathetic nervous systems." Discussion about effects of SNS stimulation can proceed.

4. Show a transparency of Table 17-1 (text, p. 212; IM, p. 137).

Clinical Laboratory

1. Ask students to assess assigned clients for signs and symptoms of SNS stimulation (stress response or "fight or flight" reaction).

2. Ask students to assess assigned clients for signs and symptoms of PNS stimulation.

TESTBANK QUESTIONS

1. An expected outcome of the administration of a beta adrenergic blocking agent is:
   a. increased cardiac output.
   b. vasodilation.
   c. bronchodilation.
   *d. decreased heart rate.

2. The following assessment is directly related to stimulation of the parasympathetic nervous system:
   a. Tachycardia
   b. Tachypnea
   *c. Bronchoconstriction
   d. Vasoconstriction

3. When anticholinergic drugs are administered, you should observe the client for:
   *a. urinary retention.
   b. diarrhea.
   c. hypotension.
   d. bradycardia.

4. Nonselective beta adrenergic blockers should be used with caution if the client has the following disorder:
   a. Peripheral vascular disease
   *b. Diabetes mellitus
   c. Tachycardia
   d. Glaucoma

5. An expected outcome after the administration of the anticholinergic drug atropine is:
   *a. increased heart rate.
   b. decreased blood pressure.
   c. decreased urinary output.
   d. increased gastric motility.

6. Beta adrenergic blockers decrease oxygen consumption of the heart by decreasing:
   *a. contractility.
   b. preload.
   c. afterload.
   d. coronary artery dilation.

7. A physiologic response to the release of acetylcholine is:
   *a. pupil constriction.
   b. decreased pulse rate.
   c. elevated blood pressure.
   d. decreased peristalsis.

8. An expected outcome after the administration of a cholinergic drug is:
   *a. bradycardia.
   b. increased platelet aggregation.
   c. peripheral dilation.
   d. increased glycogenolysis.

9. An adverse effect of the administration of beta adrenergic blockers is:
   a. headaches.
   b. tachycardia.
   c. transient chest pain.
   *d. bronchoconstriction.

10. Stimulation of the sympathetic nervous system can produce:
    a. bradycardia.
    *b. bronchodilation.
    c. coronary artery spasm.
    d. decreased surfactant production.

18
Adrenergic Drugs

MAJOR TOPICS

Adrenergic receptors
Epinephrine as the prototype of adrenergic drugs
Multipurpose adrenergic drugs

DRUG LIST

Epinephrine (Adrenalin)
Phenylephrine (Neo-Synephrine)
Phenylpropanolamine (Propagest, Accutrim, others)
Pseudoephedrine (Sudafed, others)

OBJECTIVES

1. Differentiate effects of stimulation of alpha and beta adrenergic receptors.
2. List characteristics of adrenergic drugs in terms of effects on body tissues, indications for use, adverse effects, nursing process implications, principles of therapy, and observation of client responses.
3. Discuss use of epinephrine to treat anaphylactic shock, acute bronchospasm, and cardiac arrest.

4. Identify clients at high risk of experiencing adverse effects with adrenergic drugs.
5. List commonly used OTC preparations that contain adrenergic drugs.

TEACHING STRATEGIES

Classroom

1. Discuss common conditions for which adrenergic drugs are used.

2. Ask students about their experiences with conditions for which the drugs are used.

3. Discuss review questions 3, 5, and 7 (text, p. 225).

4. Assign the Critical Thinking Case Study (SG, p. 67).

Clinical Laboratory

1. Show students the emergency drug supply. Have students select or name the adrenergic drugs and describe their preparation and administration in specific emergency situations, such as anaphylactic shock or cardiopulmonary resuscitation.

2. For clients receiving an adrenergic drug, have students assess for therapeutic and adverse effects.

3. For clients receiving an adrenergic drug, have students assess for conditions that may be aggravated by adrenergic drugs. If such conditions are found, assign students to teach the clients to avoid OTC appetite suppressants, asthma remedies (bronchodilators), nasal decongestants, and multisymptom cold remedies containing decongestants.

TESTBANK QUESTIONS

1. Epinephrine (Adrenalin) is used to:
   *a. increase the heart rate.
   b. decrease insulin secretion.
   c. increase the rate of blood coagulation.
   d. decrease fatty acid metabolism.

2. Epinephrine (Adrenalin) increases blood pressure by:
   a. increasing the production of renin.
   *b. producing vasoconstriction of peripheral vessels.
   c. decreasing urinary output.
   d. promoting the release of ADH.

3. Epinephrine (Adrenalin) cannot be administered:
   a. by inhalation.
   b. topically.
   c. parenterally.
   *d. orally.

4. If isoproterenol (Isuprel) is used for bronchospasm, an expected adverse response would be:
   a. hypotension.
   b. hyperactive reflexes.
   *c. tachycardia.
   d. dizziness.

5. With excessive use of nasal decongestants, the following can occur:
   a. Dehydration
   *b. Rebound nasal congestion
   c. Tremors
   d. Anxiety

6. A client tells you about pink-tinged respiratory secretions after receiving nebulizer treatments with isoproterenol (Isuprel). What will you do?
   a. Contact the physician immediately.
   b. Send a sputum specimen to the lab to be examined for blood.
   *c. Tell the client that this harmless coloration is due to the medication.
   d. Question the client about foods and fluids taken for breakfast.

7. The following medication is used as a nasal decongestant and an appetite suppressant:
   a. Phenylephrine (Neo-Synephrine)
   *b. Phenylpropanolamine hydrochloride (Propagest, Dexatrim)
   c. Propylhexedrine (Benzedrex)
   d. Oxymetazoline hydrochloride (Afrin)

8. Dopamine (Intropin) is used to treat:
   a. allergic reactions.
   b. bronchoconstriction.
   *c. hypotension and shock.
   d. cardiac arrest.

9. A client is admitted with an acute asthmatic attack. Before treatment is initiated, ABGs are drawn. Her pH is 7.30, pCO_2 is 30, and pO_2 is 95. She needs to be treated for:
   a. hypoxemia.
   b. hypercarbia.
   *c. acidosis.
   d. alkalosis.

10. An expected outcome after the administration of a vasopressor drug is:
    *a. improved urinary output.
    b. increased ability to breathe.
    c. warm extremities.
    d. decreased oxygen consumption.

CRITICAL THINKING CASE STUDY

1. Dopamine is administered to increase blood pressure. Lidocaine treats ventricular dysrhythmias.

2. Vital signs will be assessed because an expected outcome of the administration of these 2 medications is increased blood pressure and absence of or decreased dysrhythmias. Urinary output will be evaluated. If cardiac output is inadequate,

renal perfusion will be decreased and urinary output will drop.

3. Dobutamine is administered to increase the force of the heart's contraction and therefore increase cardiac output. If Mr. J. responds to this medication, his systolic blood pressure will be maintained above 90 and his urinary output will be 30cc or more an hour.

4. Isuprel has a vasopressor effect, so it will increase the blood pressure and also the pulse. It can be administered intravenously via IV drip and titrated according to vital sign changes.

5. The physician could insert an intra-aortic balloon pump to increase myocardial perfusion and improve the performance of the heart.

19
Antiadrenergic Drugs

MAJOR TOPICS

Effects of beta blockers on body tissues
Use of beta adrenergic blocking agents in cardiovascular disorders

DRUG LIST

Atenolol (Tenormin)
Clonidine (Catapres)
Labetalol (Normodyne, Trandate)
Metoprolol (Lopressor)
Doxazosin (Cardura)
Propranolol (Inderal)
Terazosin (Hytrin)

OBJECTIVES

1. List characteristics of antiadrenergic drugs in terms of effects on body tissues, indications for use, nursing process implications, principles of therapy, and observation of client response.
2. Discuss alpha$_1$-adrenergic blocking agents and alpha$_2$-adrenergic agonists in terms of indications for use, adverse effects, and selected other characteristics.
3. Compare and contrast currently approved beta-adrenergic blocking agents in terms of cardioselectivity, indications for use, adverse effects, and selected other characteristics.
4. Discuss teaching needs of clients taking beta blockers.

TEACHING STRATEGIES

Classroom

1. The concept that alpha$_2$-adrenergic *agonists* (e.g., clonidine and related drugs) have *antiadrenergic* effects may be confusing. Emphasize that the drugs cause less norepinephrine to be released at presynaptic nerve endings to aid student understanding of drug action.

2. Lecture/discussion about the effects and uses of alpha$_1$-adrenergic blocking agents.

3. Show a transparency that summarizes effects of beta blockers (IM, p. 138).

4. Discuss each effect in relation to the disorders for which the drugs are used and in relation to adverse drug reactions.

5. Show transparencies of Figure 19-1 (text, p. 228; IM p. 139) and of nonselective and cardioselective beta blockers (IM, p. 140). Remind students that generic names of beta blockers end in "lol" to aid recognition.

6. Show a transparency of the cardiovascular indications for use (IM, p. 141).

7. If not assigned as homework, have students complete the true-false exercise on beta blockers (SG, p. 69). This can also be displayed as a transparency and completed by the group of students.

8. Assign groups of 4 to 6 students to prepare a teaching plan for a client starting an antiadrenergic drug.

9. Assign students to write answers to the review and application exercises (text, p. 239).

10. Assign the Critical Thinking Case Study (SG, p. 71) and discuss in class.

Clinical Laboratory

1. For a client with a clonidine transdermal patch, ask a student to:
   a. consult a drug reference about application and effects (if new to the student);
   b. interview the client about application and effects;
   c. compare the client's statements with information in the drug reference and evaluate for discrepancies;
   d. resolve any discrepancies found;
   e. and accurately apply the patch if indicated.

2. For a client taking an alpha$_1$ blocker, have a student monitor blood pressure and assess for dizziness after drug administration.

3. For a client taking a beta blocker, have a student check heart rate and evaluate whether the value obtained is a therapeutic or adverse effect.

4. Ask students how they might reply when a client on a beta blocker complains of fatigue.

5. Obtain copies of agency instruction sheets related to alpha blockers and beta blockers; discuss ways to individualize instructions for particular clients.

TESTBANK QUESTIONS

1. Beta-adrenergic blockers have a negative chronotropic effect, which results in decreased:
   *a. heart rate.
   b. muscle contraction.
   c. conduction through the AV node.
   d. blood pressure.

2. Nonselective beta-adrenergic blockers used for the treatment of hypertension should be avoided in persons with:
   a. prostatic disease.
   *b. diabetes mellitus.
   c. glaucoma.
   d. tachycardia.

3. Bodily reflexes can oppose the fall in blood pressure induced by certain antihypertensive drugs by:
   a. causing the release of renin.
   *b. causing fluid retention.
   c. increasing urinary output.
   d. decreasing gastric motility.

4. Clonidine, an antihypertensive, is also used investigationally to treat:
   a. cardiac dysrhythmias.
   b. metabolic acidosis.
   *c. alcohol withdrawal.
   d. heart failure.

5. Following a myocardial infarction, your client is placed on a beta-adrenergic blocker. Which of the following statements leads you to believe that your client understands the reason this drug was ordered? "This drug will:
   a. make my heart beat harder."
   b. increase the electrical conduction in my heart."
   *c. decrease the possibility of developing heart irregularities."
   d. increase my heart rate."

6. Beta-adrenergic blockers used to treat glaucoma work by:
   *a. decreasing the formation of aqueous humor.
   b. increasing the outflow of aqueous humor.
   c. reducing the volume of vitreous humor.
   d. constricting the optic blood vessels.

7. The following is a selective beta-adrenergic blocker:
   a. Sotalol (Betapace)
   b. Timolol (Blocadren)
   c. Nadolol (Corgard)
   *d. Atenolol (Tenormin)

8. The advantage of a selective beta-adrenergic blocker over a nonselective beta-adrenergic blocker is that:
   a. it only needs to be taken once a day.
   *b. there are few respiratory problems associated with selective agents.
   c. there is a limited chance of heart failure.
   d. drug doses are significantly less.

9. Lipid-soluble beta-adrenergic blockers are more likely to cause the following adverse effects:
   *a. Confusion, hallucinations, and insomnia
   b. Hypotension and tachycardia
   c. Fatigue and dizziness
   d. Sweating, palpitations, and elevated blood sugar

10. An expected outcome when an alpha-adrenergic blocking agent is administered to a client with Raynaud's disease is:
    *a. improved skin color and temperature.
    b. increased mobility.
    c. decreased pain.
    d. decreased joint swelling.

11. Class II antidysrhythmic drugs affect the heart by:
    a. increasing cardiac blood flow.
    b. enhancing contractility of cardiac muscle.
    c. suppressing depolarization in cardiac cells.
    *d. decreasing automaticity and increasing the refractory period.

12. Which adverse effect is commonly associated with the use of beta-adrenergic blockers?
    a. Visual disturbances
    b. Hypersalivation
    c. Peripheral edema
    *d. Postural hypotension

13. A client receiving propranolol (Inderal) and a calcium channel blocker should be assessed for:
    a. chest pain.
    *b. slow pulse rate.
    c. confusion.
    d. decreased white blood count.

14. The effect on the ECG that the nurse may see when a client is receiving beta-adrenergic blockers is:
    a. sinus tachycardia.
    *b. prolonged PR interval.
    c. depressed ST segment.
    d. widened QRS complexes.

15. Esmolol (Brevibloc) is used to treat unresponsive:
    a. heart block.
    b. atrial fibrillation.
    c. ventricular tachycardia.
    *d. paroxysmal supraventricular tachycardia.

16. An expected outcome after the administration of beta-adrenergic blockers is:
    a. decreased respiratory rate.
    *b. decreased heart rate.
    c. increased urinary output.
    d. increased blood pressure.

17. Mr. J. was placed on propranolol (Inderal) for hypertension. He is complaining of impotence; what is the best response to give him?
    a. "You need to seek the advice of a sex therapist."
    *b. "Talk to your doctor; there are other medications that he can prescribe."
    c. "This is common when you first start taking this drug; it will improve."
    d. "If you want to keep your blood pressure under control, you must continue to take this medication."

20
Cholinergic Drugs

MAJOR TOPICS

Clinical uses and limitations of cholinergic drugs

DRUG LIST

Bethanechol (Urecholine)
Neostigmine (Prostigmin)

OBJECTIVES

1. Describe effects and indications for use of selected cholinergic drugs.
2. Discuss drug therapy of myasthenia gravis.
3. Discuss atropine as an antidote for cholinergic drugs.
4. Describe major nursing care needs of clients receiving cholinergic drugs.

TEACHING STRATEGIES

Classroom

1. Because these drugs are infrequently used in most settings, the instructor may choose to assign portions of the chapter to be studied independently, to emphasize a few main points in lecture, or to prepare a written handout that summarizes drug effects.

2. Discuss the prevalence of Alzheimer's disease, the limitations of current drug therapy, and the need for effective drugs.

Clinical Laboratory

1. For a client who has had thoracic or abdominal surgery, ask a student to check the operative record for administration of a cholinergic agent used to reverse effects of a neuromuscular blocking agent.

2. For a client with myasthenia gravis, ask a student to list the cholinergic drug, evaluate the dose in relation to literature recommendations, and interview the client about signs and symptoms of too much or too little drug.

3. For a client with Alzheimer's disease who is receiving donepezil or tacrine, assess the client or interview caregivers about therapeutic and adverse drug effects.

TESTBANK QUESTIONS

1. Edrophonium (Tensilon) is used to diagnose myasthenia gravis. Which antidote should be on hand when the test is performed?
   *a. Atropine
   b. Ambenonium (Mytelase)
   c. Physostigmine salicylate (Antilirium)
   d. Pyridostigmine (Mestinon)

2. Treatment of a cholinergic crisis includes withdrawal of the anticholinesterase drug and administration of:
   *a. atropine.
   b. belladonna.
   c. carbamazepine (Tegretol).
   d. phenytoin (Dilantin).

3. Your client is being treated with an anticholinesterase drug for myasthenia gravis. Which of the following indicates an improvement in his condition?
   a. Decreased pulse and increased respiratory rate
   b. Increased appetite and weight gain
   c. Decreased serum calcium levels
   *d. Increased ability to speak and swallow

4. Excessive doses of cholinergic agents can produce a cholinergic crisis. Which of the following should be reported to the physician?
   *a. Muscle weakness
   b. Absent bowel sounds
   c. Hypertension
   d. Absent deep tendon reflexes

5. Anticholinesterase drugs:
   a. decrease respiratory secretions.
   b. dilate pupils.
   c. decrease salivary gland secretions.
   *d. improve skeletal muscle contraction.

6. Mr. H. has postoperative hypoperistalsis, and his physician orders bethanechol (Urecholine). In addition to the medication, what other nursing action would be beneficial?
   a. Medicate him for pain
   b. Force fluids
   *c. Ambulate Mr. H. in the hall
   d. Apply a heating pad to his abdomen

7. After her morning dose of ambenonium (Mytelase), your client begins to have difficulty breathing. Identify your nursing actions:
   a. Encourage her to turn, cough, and deep breathe
   *b. Contact her physician immediately
   c. Assess her O$_2$ saturation
   d. Determine her respiratory rate and blood pressure

8. Pyridostigmine (Mestinon) is to be administered 3 times per day. The best schedule for administration of this drug is:
   a. 8 a.m., 12 p.m., 4 p.m.
   b. 9 a.m., 3 p.m., 9 p.m.
   c. 8 a.m., 2 p.m., 12 a.m.
   *d. 6 a.m., 2 p.m., 10 p.m.

9. After receiving bethanechol (Urecholine), your client's BP drops to 86/60. You should:
   a. know that a drop in BP is common with this drug.
   *b. notify her physician.
   c. check her BP every hour for the next 4 hours.
   d. have her walk in the hall and then check her BP again.

10. Following general anesthesia, the following medication can be used to reverse neuromuscular blockade:
    a. Bethanechol (Urecholine)
    *b. Neostigmine (Prostigmin)
    c. Edrophonium (Tensilon)
    d. Physostigmine salicylate (Antilirium)

11. Neostigmine (Prostigmin) is ordered for your client's urinary retention. Which of the following medications should you report to Mr. B.'s physician before giving the neostigmine?
    *a. Antihistamine
    b. Anti-inflammatory agent
    c. Antidiabetic agent
    d. Antidepressant

12. M.J. weighs 66 lbs. Her physician orders pyridostigmine (Mestinon) 2 mg/kg q8h. How much will you administer per day?
    a. 360 mg
    b. 120 mg
    *c. 180 mg
    d. 240 mg

CRITICAL THINKING CASE STUDY

1. J. has undergone abdominal surgery, during which he received general anesthesia, which decreases bowel function. His bowel was also manipulated during the procedure. His bowel sounds should return in 24–48 hours. Activity usually enhances the return of bowel sounds.

2. J.'s NG tube is suctioning hydrochloric acid out of his stomach, which can cause alkalosis and hypokalemia.

3. The physician ordered Urecholine to increase tone and contractility of gastrointestinal and bladder smooth muscle. The recommended pediatric dose is .1 mg/kg and may be increased up to .4 mg/kg every 4 hours. J. weighs 30 kilograms. Therefore the recommended dose would be 3 mg.

4. J. should have decreased abdominal distention, audible bowel sounds, and be able to void adequate amounts of urine without difficulty.

5. Hypotension, miosis, and increased perspiration are adverse effects of cholinergic drugs. The nurse should also assess J. for symptoms of infection because J. is tachycardic and his temperature is elevated. The next dose of Urecholine should be held, and his physician should be contacted.

6. A cholinergic crisis can precipitate respiratory failure. Atropine is the antidote for cholinergic agents.

21
Anticholinergic Drugs

MAJOR TOPICS

Effects of anticholinergic drugs on body tissues
Indications and limitations on clinical use of anticholinergic drugs

DRUG LIST

Atropine sulfate
Glycopyrrolate (Robinul)

OBJECTIVES

1. List characteristics of anticholinergic drugs in terms of effects on body tissues, indications for use, nursing process implications, observation of client responses, and teaching clients.
2. Discuss atropine as the prototype of anticholinergic drugs.
3. Discuss clinical disorders/symptoms for which anticholinergic drugs are used.
4. Describe the mechanism by which atropine relieves bradycardia.
5. Review anticholinergic effects of antipsychotics, tricyclic antidepressants, and antihistamines.

TEACHING STRATEGIES

Classroom

1. Review selected effects of acetylcholine.
2. Explain that the effects of anticholinergic drugs stem directly from their ability to block acetylcholine receptors in various body tissues.
3. Discuss the Critical Thinking Case Study (SG, p. 77).

Clinical Laboratory

1. For clients receiving one or more drugs with anticholinergic effects, have students assess for therapeutic and adverse drug effects.

2. Discuss nursing interventions that prevent or decrease dry mouth, urinary retention, and tachycardia associated with systemic anticholinergic drugs.

TESTBANK QUESTIONS

1. Your client is to begin trihexyphenidyl (Artane). Which of the following conditions would contraindicate its use?
   a. Hemoglobin of 11 g/dl
   b. Blood glucose of 180 mg/dl
   c. Blood pressure of 90/60
   *d. Pulse of 110

2. Clients who are taking anticholinergic medications should avoid the concurrent use of:
   a. aspirin products.
   *b. antihistamines.
   c. antacids.
   d. acetaminophen.

3. Anticholinergic drugs are administered to clients with Parkinson's disease to decrease:
   *a. tremors.
   b. ataxia.
   c. slurred speech.
   d. difficulty swallowing.

4. Which of the following disorders in Mr. H.'s history should you make the physician aware of before giving procyclidine (Kemadrin)?
   a. Asthma
   *b. Benign prostatic hypertrophy
   c. Colon cancer
   d. Hyperlipidemia

5. The nurse should be aware that the use of anticholinergic medications can increase:
   a. acne.
   b. blood urea nitrogen levels.
   c. cataract formation.
   *d. esophageal reflux.

6. Which of the following assessments should the nurse perform prior to the administration of an anticholinergic medication for enuresis?
   a. Mental status
   b. Skin turgor
   c. Bladder function
   *d. Bowel function

7. Which of the following anticholinergic medications is administered for its bronchodilating effects?
   a. Anisotropine (Valpin)
   *b. Ipratropium (Atrovent)
   c. Dicyclomine hydrochloride (Bentyl)
   d. Methscopolamine (Pamine)

8. An expected outcome after the administration of flavoxate (Urispas) is decreased:
   a. cough.
   b. weakness.
   c. constipation.
   *d. frequency of urination.

9. The physician orders 0.25 mg of atropine for 3-year-old M.J. Atropine comes in a vial with .04 mg/ml. How many ml will you administer?
   a. 0.2 ml
   b. 0.4 ml
   *c. 0.6 ml
   d. 0.8 ml

10. Adverse effects associated with the use of anticholinergic medications include increased:
   *a. intraocular pressure.
   b. sweating.
   c. gastric motility.
   d. respiratory rate.

11. Which of the following statements by Mrs. J. leads you to believe that she has understood the teaching that you have done regarding methantheline bromide (Banthine). "This medication will:
   a. help heal my peptic ulcer."
   *b. help relieve my abdominal pain."
   c. cure my intestinal infection."
   d. control my diarrhea."

12. The following medication is used to treat the extrapyramidal symptoms caused by antipsychotic drugs:
   *a. Benztropine (Cogentin)
   b. Flavoxate (Urispas)
   c. Methscopolamine (Pamine)
   d. Homatropine methylbromide (Homapin)

CRITICAL THINKING CASE STUDY

1. The confusion could be a reaction to the atropine. The nurse should perform a complete assessment, including assessing vital signs, lab values (creatinine, digoxin levels, electrolytes, hemoglobin), O_2 saturation, and neurological checks, to help determine the cause of the confusion. The physician should be made aware of the change in the client's status.

2. The dry mouth and blurred vision are related to administration of atropine and will subside.

3. A pacemaker treats electrical conduction failure and causes the heart to beat at a regular rate, but it does not cure heart failure. Mr. P. will probably continue to take medications for his heart failure.

IV
DRUGS AFFECTING THE ENDOCRINE SYSTEM

22
Physiology of the Endocrine System

MAJOR TOPICS
Endocrine organs
Endocrine–nervous system interactions
General characteristics of hormones

OBJECTIVES
1. Discuss the relationship between the endocrine system and the central nervous system (CNS).
2. Describe general characteristics and functions of hormones.
3. Differentiate steroid and protein hormones in relation to site of action and pharmacokinetics.
4. Discuss hormonal action at the cellular level.
5. Describe the second-messenger roles of cyclic adenosine monophosphate (cAMP) and calcium within body cells.
6. Differentiate between physiologic and pharmacologic doses of hormonal drugs.

TEACHING STRATEGIES

Classroom
1. Ask students to define "hormone" and ask additional questions to determine what students already know about hormones.
2. Discuss review and application exercises 2 and 4 (text, p. 265).

Clinical Laboratory
1. Have students identify and assess assigned clients for hormone imbalance.
2. For a client receiving a hormonal drug, ask students to determine whether the dose is physiologic or pharmacologic.

TESTBANK QUESTIONS

1. Thyroid hormones:
   a. raise blood glucose levels by promoting hepatic glycogenolysis.
   *b. are necessary for growth and development in children.
   c. regulate osmolality of extracellular fluid.
   d. are necessary for protein metabolism.

2. When a female ovulates, increased amounts of this hormone are available:
   a. Epinephrine
   b. Insulin
   *c. Estrogen
   d. Thyroxine

3. A client is admitted with weight gain, lethargy, and bradycardia. Based on these symptoms, you would suspect an abnormality in which of the following endocrine glands?
   a. Adrenal
   *b. Thyroid
   c. Pancreas
   d. Parathyroid

4. M.A., a 6 year old, is diagnosed with diabetes mellitus. Her physician prescribes insulin because adequate insulin levels are necessary for:
   *a. normal growth and development.
   b. development of secondary sex characteristics.
   c. regulation of red blood cell production.
   d. elimination of sugar from the body.

5. ADH is secreted by the pituitary in response to low:
   a. serum sodium levels.
   *b. blood volume.
   c. specific gravity.
   d. serum glucose levels.

6. The parathyroid hormone:
   a. promotes potassium retention and sodium excretion.
   b. regulates metabolism of glucose, lipids, and proteins.
   *c. regulates calcium and phosphorus metabolism.
   d. promotes carbohydrate storage and protein catabolism.

7. The following hormone, secreted by the gastric mucosa, is important in the digestive process:
   a. Liothyronine
   *b. Cholecystokinin
   c. Tetraiodothyronine
   d. Gastrin

8. Corticosteroids are administered for the treatment of:
   *a. acute respiratory disorders.
   b. acne.
   c. angina.
   d. alcohol withdrawal.

9. This synthetic hormone is administered to persons in end-stage renal failure (ESRF) to stimulate RBC production:
   a. Enterogastrone
   b. Epinephrine
   *c. Erythropoietin
   d. Secretin

10. Addison's disease is treated with:
    *a. adrenal corticosteroids.
    b. parathyroid hormones.
    c. thyroid hormones.
    d. progesterone.

11. Persons receiving corticosteroids need to be monitored for increases in:
    *a. weight.
    b. potassium levels.
    c. secondary sex characteristics.
    d. red blood cell production.

23
Hypothalamic and Pituitary Hormones

MAJOR TOPICS
Hypothalamus and its secretions
Pituitary gland and its secretions

DRUG LIST
Growth hormone (Somatrem, Somatropin)
Oxytocin (Pitocin)

OBJECTIVES
1. Describe clinical uses of major pituitary hormones.
2. Differentiate characteristics and functions of anterior and posterior pituitary hormones.
3. Discuss limitations of hypothalamic and pituitary hormones as therapeutic agents.
4. State major nursing considerations in the care of clients receiving specific hypothalamic and pituitary hormones.

TEACHING STRATEGIES

Classroom

1. Discuss reasons for infrequent use of hypothalamic and pituitary hormones in clinical practice.

2. Discuss growth hormone as an example of a hormone affecting essentially all body cells.

3. Describe characteristics of a young child that may indicate inadequate endogenous growth hormone.

Clinical Laboratory

1. In a medical-surgical setting, discuss the advantages of administering an adrenal corticosteroid rather than corticotropin (ACTH).

2. In an obstetric setting, review the dose, route, and specific monitoring of a client receiving oxytocin to induce or augment the labor process.

TESTBANK QUESTIONS

1. A client with diabetes insipidus is to receive lypressin. The route of administration will be:
   a. oral.
   b. intramuscular.
   c. intravenous.
   *d. intranasal.

2. Two hours after administering vasopressin (Pitressin), your client complains of a throbbing headache. This symptom is:
   a. due to a subtherapeutic dose and you should administer another dose.
   b. an allergic reaction and you should administer Benadryl.
   c. a toxic effect and you should contact the physician immediately.
   *d. a common adverse effect due to vasoconstriction; continue to assess.

3. The physician orders 10 units of oxytocin (Pitocin) in 1000 ml of D5W (10 milliunits/ml). Using microdrip tubing (1 ml = 60 drops), how fast will you run the IV to administer 2 milliunits/minute?
   a. 11 drops/minute
   *b. 12 drops/minute
   c. 13 drops/minute
   d. 15 drops/minute

4. An expected urinary output when lypressin is administered for diabetes insipidus is:
   a. 30 cc/hour.
   *b. 1500–2000 cc/24 hours.
   c. 200 cc/hour for 24 hours.
   d. 4000–5000 cc/24 hours.

5. Before administering somatropin (Humatrope) to a 7 year old with a deficiency of endogenous growth hormone, you should verify:
   a. adequate renal function.
   b. the child's ability to understand the treatment.
   *c. evidence of open bone epiphyses.
   d. allergies to shell fish.

6. Menotropins (Pergonal), used to induce ovulation, contains the following hormone(s):
   a. Corticotropin and somatotropin
   *b. Luteinizing hormone and follicle stimulating hormone
   c. Gonadotropin-releasing hormone
   d. Thyrotropin-releasing hormone

CRITICAL THINKING CASE STUDY

1. This medication will increase the force of your contractions and help your labor progress.

2. There must be continuous monitoring of uterine contractions, fetal and maternal heart rates, and maternal blood pressure and respiratory rate. The physician should be notified if contractions last longer than 1 minute or occur more frequently than every 2 minutes. Intake and output should also be monitored.

3. The Pitocin is increased slowly to allow for a gradual increase in uterine contractions.

4. Encourage Ms. G. to use the relaxation techniques she learned during prenatal classes. Contact her physician to see if he will allow her to have pain medications.

5. Pitocin is continued after delivery for many individuals to control uterine bleeding.

24
Corticosteroids

MAJOR TOPICS

Effects of endogenous corticosteroids on body function and metabolism
Use and effects of exogenous corticosteroids

DRUG LIST

Beclomethasone (Beclovent, Vanceril, Vancenase)
Dexamethasone (Decadron)
Fluticasone (Flonase)
Hydrocortisone
Methylprednisolone (Medrol, others)
Prednisone
Triamcinolone (Azmacort)

OBJECTIVES

1. Review physiologic effects of endogenous corticosteroids.

2. List at least five clinical indications for use of exogenous corticosteroids.
3. Differentiate between physiologic and pharmacologic doses of corticosteroids.
4. Differentiate between short-term and long-term corticosteroid therapy.
5. List at least ten adverse effects of long-term corticosteroid therapy.
6. Explain the pathophysiologic basis of adverse effects.
7. State the rationale for giving corticosteroids topically when possible rather than systemically.
8. Use other drugs and interventions to decrease the need for corticosteroids.
9. Apply the nursing process with a client receiving long-term corticosteroid therapy, including teaching needs.

TEACHING STRATEGIES

Classroom

1. Because of the importance and frequent clinical use of these drugs, this content warrants one or two class periods.

2. The objectives may be used as an outline for lecture/discussion. Discuss hydrocortisone as the prototypical drug and the others as commonly used drugs in a variety of clinical settings.

3. Emphasize that many corticosteroids are available in several different formulations, for various indications and routes of administration. These formulations are not interchangeable and should be used solely for the designated purpose or route.

4. Ask students to share their previous experiences with clients receiving corticosteroids.

5. Show a transparency of the worksheet on adverse effects (SG, p. 87) and complete it with student input and discussion.

6. Assign the Critical Thinking Case Study (SG, p. 89) as homework to be turned in. This will assist in evaluating student understanding of corticosteroid therapy.

Clinical Laboratory

1. Have students administer corticosteroids by oral, intravenous, inhalation, and topical routes when opportunities arise. In clinical conferences, discuss advantages and disadvantages of various routes.

2. For clients receiving a corticosteroid drug, discuss the reason for use and the expected effects in each client.

3. For clients on long-term corticosteroid therapy, have students assess for edema, increased blood pressure, bruised skin, hypokalemia, hyperglycemia, and other adverse effects.

4. Review agency instruction sheets for various corticosteroids and ask students to individualize them for assigned clients.

TESTBANK QUESTIONS

1. Prednisone antagonizes the effect of vitamin D and thereby decreases the intestinal absorption of:
   a. sodium
   b. potassium
   *c. calcium
   d. magnesium

2. An insulin-dependent diabetic is started on prednisone (Deltasone). Which of the following statements leads you to believe that he has understood the teaching you have done? "I will need to:
   a. decrease the amount of insulin I am taking."
   *b. increase the amount of insulin I am taking."
   c. keep my insulin dosage the same."
   d. stop taking my insulin while I am receiving this medication."

3. Postmenopausal women taking corticosteroids to prevent osteoporosis should:
   *a. exercise.
   b. drink 4 glasses of milk a day.
   c. eat foods high in vitamin K.
   d. take the medication with antacids.

4. Prednisone is given to a 5-year-old child with nephrosis to:
   a. cause diuresis.
   b. prevent sodium retention.
   *c. reduce urinary protein loss.
   d. suppress infection.

5. With which of the following diseases should corticosteroids be administered with caution?
   a. Peripheral vascular disease
   b. Prostatic hypertrophy
   c. Chronic obstructive pulmonary disease
   *d. Peptic ulcer disease

6. Corticosteroid inhalers are administered to:
   a. produce bronchodilation.
   *b. decrease inflammation.
   c. prevent the release of histamine.
   d. decrease the respiratory rate.

7. G.P., age 9, is receiving prednisone (Deltasone) along with other immunosuppressants to prevent rejection of his newly transplanted lung. It is important for you to inform G.P.'s parents of the following:
   *a. Stunting of growth can occur with long-term steroid use.
   b. Long-term steroid use can prevent development of secondary sex characteristics.
   c. Long-term steroid use can cause weight loss.
   d. Alopecia can occur with long-term steroid use.

8. A client with multiple sclerosis being treated with adrenocorticotropic hormone (ACTH) should be instructed to:
   a. restrict fluid intake to 2 liters per day.
   b. purchase a wig because alopecia may occur.
   *c. include foods high in potassium.
   d. use aspirin for minor discomforts.

9. Corticosteroids should be administered with caution to clients with the following disorder:
   a. Asthma
   b. Chronic lung disease
   *c. Diabetes mellitus
   d. Crohn's disease

10. Oral corticosteroids administered for extended periods of time can cause:
    a. calcium to be reabsorbed.
    b. chloride to be reabsorbed.
    *c. potassium to be excreted.
    d. sodium to be excreted.

11. Your client has been started on beclomethasone (Vanceril) and albuterol (Proventil) inhalers. You know that your teaching has been successful if he states:
    a. "I may gain weight from taking these medications."
    b. "I will take these medications with meals to prevent nausea."
    c. "I will roll the inhalers gently between my hands before administering them."
    *d. "I will use the Proventil first, then the Vanceril."

CRITICAL THINKING CASE STUDY

1. G.'s mother should be aware of G.'s nutritional needs. She may need to increase the K^+ and Ca^{++} in his diet. G. will have an increased appetite, so she will need to provide low-calorie snacks to prevent excessive weight gain. Corticosteroid use can cause growth retardation, and G.'s mother needs to know this. Hyperglycemia is an adverse effect of the medication, so his blood sugar will need to be monitored routinely. G. will also be more susceptible to infection, so G.'s mother needs to monitor any cuts or abrasions and observe for any symptoms of infection.

2. At this point there is no way of knowing how long the treatment will be.

3. It would probably be helpful for her son to talk to a counselor about his feelings. If there is another child who he could talk to with the same condition that may also be helpful. Encourage G.'s mother to ask the physician for information regarding the length of treatment. G. may also need to be on a stricter diet with daily exercise.

25
Thyroid and Antithyroid Drugs

MAJOR TOPICS
Effects of thyroid disorders on body systems

DRUG LIST
Levothyroxine (Synthroid)
Propylthiouracil (Propacil)

OBJECTIVES
1. Describe physiologic effects of thyroid hormone.
2. Identify effects of hypo- and hypersecretion of thyroid hormone.
3. Describe characteristics, uses, and effects of thyroid drugs.
4. Describe characteristics, uses, and effects of antithyroid drugs.
5. Discuss the influence of thyroid and antithyroid drugs on the metabolism of other drugs.
6. Teach clients self-care activities related to the use of thyroid and antithyroid drugs.

TEACHING STRATEGIES

Classroom

1. Review the role of thyroid hormone in body metabolism.

2. Use Table 25-1 (text, p. 297) to demonstrate the generally opposing effects of hypo- and hyper-thyroidism.

3. Emphasize that drug therapy of one disorder may cause the other disorder.

4. Use the Critical Thinking Case Study (SG, p. 93) as a basis for class discussion, or assign it for small group discussions.

Clinical Laboratory

1. For a client receiving levothyroxine or propylthiouracil, have a student assess for signs and symptoms of the disorder being treated (to evaluate therapeutic affects) and for the opposing disorder (to evaluate adverse effects).

2. Review laboratory reports of assigned clients for thyroid function tests (e.g., TSH, T_3, T_4).

TESTBANK QUESTIONS

1. A client with weight loss, insomnia, and tachycardia is diagnosed with hyperthyroidism. The drug of choice for treating the tachycardia is:
   *a. propranolol (Inderal).
   b. digoxin (Lanoxin).
   c. verapamil (Calan).
   d. quinidine.

2. The following is used to adjust levothyroxine (Synthroid) doses:
   a. Serum total thyroxine test
   *b. Serum thyroid-stimulating hormone (TSH) test
   c. Serum iodide
   d. Free thyroxine index

3. Levothyroxine (Synthroid) is commonly administered:
   *a. q.d.
   b. t.i.d.
   c. q.o.d
   d. b.i.d.

4. A client receiving levothyroxine (Synthroid) needs to be assessed for hyperthyroidism, symptoms of which include:
   a. cold, dry, scaly skin.
   b. slow cognitive ability.
   c. depression.
   *d. fine tremor and weight loss.

5. A 7 year old has been diagnosed with hypothyroidism. If she remains untreated, the following will occur:
   *a. growth retardation.
   b. renal dysfunction.
   c. increased bowel movements and diarrhea.
   d. malnutrition.

6. Sodium iodine, used for the treatment of hyperthyroidism, should not be administered to:
   a. elderly individuals.
   b. middle-aged women with osteoporosis.
   *c. pregnant women.
   d. children under the age of 21.

CRITICAL THINKING CASE STUDY

1. The symptoms attributable to hyperthyroidism include: weight loss, tachycardia, insomnia, and excessive perspiration.

2. Propylthiouracil (Propacil) is used to treat hyperthyroidism. Its therapeutic effect may not occur for days or weeks because of stored hormones. She will take the medication until her hyperthyroidism has been effectively treated. Propranolol (Inderal) is used for Mrs. G.'s tachycardia. She can begin to see therapeutic effects within 24–48 hours. It will be used to control tachycardia until the hyperthyroid symptoms are controlled.

3. When you are taking propylthiouracil (Propacil), you should observe for: hypothyroidism, blood disorders, skin rashes, headache, dizziness, drowsiness, nausea, vomiting, abdominal discomfort, edema, joint pain, and drug fever. Inderal can cause hypotension, bronchospasm, dizziness, fatigue, depression, insomnia, and hallucinations. Since Mrs. G. was already having problems with insomnia, she should contact her physician if her insomnia does not get better or gets worse.

4. Hypothyroidism must be treated because it decreases all the functions of the body. The cardiovascular effects include: decreased cardiac output, decreased heart rate, and heart failure.

5. Instruct Mrs. G. to take the medication as directed and not to discontinue it without consulting her physician. She should be instructed on how to check her pulse, and she should notify her physician if her resting pulse stays above 100 bpm or drops below 60 bpm. Advise her to notify her physician if headache, nervousness, diarrhea, excessive sweating, heat intolerance, chest pain, increased pulse rate, palpitations, weight loss > 2 lbs. per week, or any unusual symptoms occur. Caution her to avoid taking other medications unless instructed by her physician. Instruct her to inform any other physicians or dentists of her thyroid therapy. Emphasize the importance of follow-up exams.

26
Hormones That Regulate Calcium and Phosphorus Metabolism

MAJOR TOPICS

Parathyroid hormone, calcitonin, and vitamin D
Calcium and phosphorus functions, requirements, and sources
Drugs for hypocalcemia and hypercalcemia

DRUG LIST

Calcitonin-human (Cibacalcin)
Calcium carbonate (Os-Cal, Tums)
Calcium chloride
Calcitriol (Rocaltrol)
Etidronate (Didronel)
Gallium (Ganite)

OBJECTIVES

1. Describe the roles of parathyroid hormone, calcitonin, and vitamin D in regulating calcium metabolism.
2. Identify populations at risk of developing hypocalcemia.
3. Discuss prevention and treatment of hypocalcemia.
4. Identify clients at risk of developing hypercalcemia.
5. Discuss recognition and management of hypercalcemia as a medical emergency.

TEACHING STRATEGIES

Classroom

1. Ask students about their personal intake of calcium (e.g., use of dairy products) and to evaluate personal intake in relation to recommended dietary intake.

2. Discuss reasons for adolescent and young adult women being considered high risk groups for inadequate dietary intake of calcium.

3. Discuss ways for high risk groups to increase their intake of calcium.

4. Assign the Critical Thinking Case Study (SG, p. 97) for small group or class discussion.

Clinical Laboratory

1. Have students assess clients in relation to their risks of developing hypocalcemia or hypercalcemia.

2. Have students list serum calcium levels from their patients' medical records and evaluate these in terms of implications for nursing care.

3. Review emergency drugs located in the clinical setting and determine which may be used in treating hypocalcemia or hypercalcemia.

4. For a patient receiving chemotherapy for cancer, review serum calcium reports and evaluate his or her risks of developing hypercalcemia.

TESTBANK QUESTIONS

1. The following is a function of calcium in the body:
   a. Generation of action potential
   *b. Contraction of skeletal muscle, smooth muscle, and cardiac muscle
   c. Enables the influx of sodium in excitable tissues
   d. All of the above

2. The parathyroid hormone increases serum calcium levels by:
   a. increasing bone breakdown and release of calcium.
   b. stimulating renal tubular reabsorption of calcium.
   c. stimulating absorption of calcium from food.
   *d. all of the above.

3. A primary function of extracellular phosphorus is:
   a. activation of B-complex vitamins.
   *b. acid-base buffering.
   c. carbohydrate metabolism.
   d. protein metabolism.

4. The following food contains the *most* calcium:
   a. Whole milk (8 oz)
   b. Cheddar cheese (1 cup)
   *c. Low-fat yogurt (1 cup)
   d. Raw Broccoli (1/2 cup)

5. The following is a complication of hypocalcemia:
   a. Decreased level of consciousness progressing to unresponsiveness
   *b. Muscle tetany progressing to seizures
   c. Bradycardia progressing to cardiac failure
   d. Hypoventilation progressing to respiratory arrest

6. The following is a nursing responsibility during the infusion of calcium chloride:
   a. Administer the infusion as quickly as tolerated.
   *b. Assess for Chvostek's and Trousseau's signs regularly.
   c. Assess the infusion site every 4 hours for signs of infiltration.
   d. Continuously monitor the respiratory status.

7. The following is a biologic response to hypercalcemia:
   *a. Decreased nerve and muscle function.
   b. Decrease in clotting times
   c. Increase in bone density
   d. All of the above

8. The following medication is useful in treating hypercalcemia:
   a. Hydrochlorothiazide (HydroDIURIL)
   b. Phenytoin (Dilantin)
   *c. Furosemide (Lasix)
   d. Kayexalate

9. Administration of the following medication will lower serum calcium levels over time.
   *a. Prednisone
   b. Vitamin E
   c. Spironolactone (Aldactone)
   d. Phenobarbital

10. Mrs. H. is admitted for uncontrolled diabetes. The nurse should observe her for symptoms of the following electrolyte imbalances:
    a. Hypokalemia
    b. Hypocalcemia
    *c. Hypercalcemia
    d. Hyperphosphatemia

11. Calcitonin is used for clients with renal disease to:
    *a. decrease movement of calcium from bone to serum.
    b. interfere with calcium metabolism.
    c. decrease renal excretion of calcium.
    d. increase the production of calcium.

12. A deficiency of vitamin D:
    a. decreases parathyroid function.
    b. increases the excretion of calcium and phosphorus.
    c. leads to renal failure.
    *d. causes inadequate absorption of calcium and phosphorus.

13. Calcium is necessary for:
    a. maintaining acid-base balance.
    *b. transmission of nerve impulses.
    c. use of glucose and production of energy.
    d. proper function of B vitamins.

14. Clinical manifestation(s) of hypocalcemia include:
    *a. numbness and tingling of fingers and toes.
    b. weakness and ataxia.
    c. frequent epistaxis.
    d. ischemia of the extremities.

15. Hypocalcemia is associated with:
    a. a vegetarian diet.
    b. anticoagulants.
    c. antacid therapy.
    *d. lactose intolerance.

16. The following statement by a client receiving a vitamin D preparation leads you to believe that he has understood the teaching you have done:
    a. "I will avoid going out in the sun."
    *b. "This is a fat soluble vitamin, so it can accumulate."
    c. "I will minimize my intake of calcium now that I am taking this vitamin."
    d. "No longer can I take over-the-counter medication."

17. You are teaching a client who will be taking a calcium supplement. You should include the following information:
    a. "Take the calcium supplement with meals."
    b. "All the daily calcium supplement can be taken at one time if desired."
    *c. "Calcium-based antacids can be used as calcium supplements."
    d. "Liquid supplements are better absorbed than tablets."

CRITICAL THINKING CASE STUDY

1. The nurse will assess for problems associated with renal failure. The assessments include vital signs, urinary output, and weights. The nurse will also observe for symptoms of hyperkalemia and hypercalcemia, which include: abdominal cramping, muscle weakness, ECG changes, lethargy, personality changes, confusion, and paresthesia.

2. Intravenous normal saline will increase urinary calcium excretion. Concurrent administration of Lasix decreases the risk of fluid overload and enhances urinary excretion of calcium and potassium. Administration of prednisone also increases calcium and potassium loss.

3. A complete assessment will be done, including vital signs, breath sounds, and a neurological exam. After completing the physical exam, you will read the nursing notes from dialysis and look at the lab work. A big concern after dialysis is disequilibrium syndrome; if symptoms worsen, contact the dialysis nurse or physician.

4. Lasix should be administered as early in the day as possible to prevent nocturia. Electrolyte levels need to be monitored on a regular basis. Weekly weights should be taken to evaluate the effectiveness of the medication.

27
Antidiabetic Drugs

MAJOR TOPICS

Types, characteristics, and complications of diabetes
   mellitus
Types of insulin

DRUG LIST

Regular, NPH, and Lente insulins
Insulin lispro (Humalog)
Acarbose (Precose)
glipizide (Glucotrol)
glyburide (Diaβeta, Micronase)
Metformin (Glucophage)
Miglitol (Glyset)
Troglitazone (Rezulin)

OBJECTIVES

1. Describe major effects of endogenous insulin on body
   tissues.
2. Discuss regular, NPH, and Lente insulins in terms of
   indications for use, route of administration, and
   duration of action.
3. Differentiate between human insulin and animal
   insulin.
4. Discuss the relationships among diet, exercise, and
   drug therapy in controlling diabetes.
5. Recognize normal, hypoglycemic, and hyperglycemic
   levels of blood glucose.
6. Differentiate types of oral antidiabetic agents in terms
   of mechanisms of action, indications for use, adverse
   effects, client teaching, and nursing process
   implications.
7. Explain the benefits of maintaining glycemic control in
   preventing complications of diabetes.
8. State reasons for combinations of insulin and oral
   agents or two types of oral agents.
9. Teach clients how to recognize and treat
   hypoglycemic reactions.
10. Collaborate with nurse-diabetes educators, dietitians,
    and others in teaching self-care activities to clients
    with diabetes.

TEACHING STRATEGIES

Classroom

1. This content warrants one or more class periods,
   unless drug therapy of diabetes is extensively discussed in another nursing course. The objectives
   can be used as an outline for lecture/discussion.
2. Show a transparency of Figure 27-1 (text, p. 323;
   IM, p. 142) to aid understanding of insulin
   action and glucose metabolism.
3. Discuss regular insulin as the prototype and
   other insulins as modifications of regular insulin.
   Humulin R, Humulin N, and Novolin 70/30 are
   commonly used trade names.

4. Discuss advantages and disadvantages of intensive insulin therapy.
5. Discuss types, characteristics, and differences of
   oral antidiabetic agents.
6. Discuss trends of using combinations of insulin
   and oral agents or two types of oral agents in
   treatment of type II diabetes.
7. Ask students to write out answers to the review
   and application exercises (text, p. 349) and turn
   them in. Grades, points, or credits are recommended because of the number of questions and
   the time and effort required.
8. Ask students about their experiences with diabetic family members or clients.
9. Ask a nurse-diabetes educator to speak to the
   class about assisting clients with their antidiabetic drugs and other aspects of managing diabetes.
10. Obtain patient-oriented pamphlets and newslet-
    ters from a local chapter of the American Dia-
    betes Association and circulate them among class
    members to demonstrate a community resource.
11. Discuss teaching needs in relation to diet, exer-
    cise, and antidiabetic drugs; emphasize the need
    to include family members or significant others
    in teaching sessions.
12. Assign small groups to complete portions of the
    Critical Thinking Case Study (SG, p. 100), then
    discuss as a class.

Clinical Laboratory

1. Have students measure blood glucose levels of
   themselves, other students, or clients.
2. Have students participate in teaching newly diagnosed diabetic clients and their families. Locate
   and discuss client-teaching materials available in
   a health-care setting. If available, show patient
   education videotapes related to the disease
   process, nonpharmacologic treatment measures,
   and pharmacologic treatments.
3. Have students administer insulin.
4. Have students monitor clients' laboratory reports
   for glycosylated hemoglobin levels, when available, and discuss nursing process implications of
   normal and abnormal values.
5. For clients receiving one or more antidiabetic
   drugs, ask students to assess for risk and for signs
   and symptoms of hypoglycemia.
6. Have a dietitian speak to a clinical group about
   dietary counseling with a diabetic client and family members.

TESTBANK QUESTIONS

1. Insulin injection sites may be rotated to prevent:
   a. allergic reactions.
   b. constriction of peripheral vessels.
   *c. lipodystrophy.
   d. accumulation and prolonged effect.

2. Symptoms of hypoglycemia include:
   a. tingling of extremities.
   b. polyuria and polydipsia.
   *c. headache and slurred speech.
   d. abdominal cramps and blurred vision.

3. When an insulin-dependent diabetic is started on prednisone, her insulin dose:
   a. may need to be decreased.
   *b. may need to be increased.
   c. will remain the same.
   d. will be stopped.

4. An insulin dependent diabetic starts an exercise program; his insulin will probably need to be:
   a. spread evenly throughout the day.
   b. supplemented with an oral agent.
   *c. decreased.
   d. changed to once a day.

5. The following drug can mask the symptoms of hypoglycemia:
   *a. Propranolol (Inderal)
   b. Furosemide (Lasix)
   c. Disopyramide (Norpace)
   d. Phenytoin (Dilantin)

6. Insulin:
   a. releases fatty acids for use as fuel.
   *b. promotes transport of glucose into fat cells.
   c. increases glucose transport into brain cells.
   d. breaks down glycogen.

7. The following insulin solution is the most efficient in bringing down blood glucose levels in diabetic ketoacidosis:
   a. Humulin N
   b. Novolin 70/30
   *c. Humulin R
   d. Ultralente

8. The following oral agent only needs to be administered once a day:
   a. Acetohexamide (Dymelor)
   *b. Glyburide (Micronase)
   c. Tolazamide (Tolinase)
   d. Tolbutamide (Orinase)

9. Insulin cannot be taken orally because:
   a. the onset of action is slow and prolonged.
   b. glucose levels sink too low.
   *c. enzymes in the gastrointestinal tract destroy insulin.
   d. bioavailability is hard to predict.

10. Symptoms of hypoglycemia may be severe when glucose levels drop to:
    a. 99 mg/dl.
    b. 69 mg/dl.
    *c. 39 mg/dl.
    d. 19 mg/dl.

11. Acarbose (Precose) and miglitol (Glyset) decrease blood sugar by:
    a. increasing pancreatic secretion of insulin.
    *b. slowing digestion of complex carbohydrates.
    c. inhibiting metabolism of fats and thereby reducing caloric intake.
    d. increasing tissue sensitivity to insulin.

12. Lactic acidosis is a life-threatening adverse effect that may occur with which of the following antidiabetic drugs?
    a. Glyburide (Diaβeta)
    b. Acarbose (Precose)
    *c. Metformin (Glucophage)
    d. Troglitazone (Rezulin)

13. For a client with diabetes, the nurse notes a physician's orders for glyburide (Diaβeta) and acarbose (Precose). How should the nurse proceed?
    *a. Give the drugs as ordered.
    b. Omit both drugs and ask the physician to correct an apparently erroneous order.
    c. Give the glyburide and withhold the acarbose until able to consult the prescribing physician.
    d. Give the acarbose and withhold the glyburide until able to consult the prescribing physician.

CRITICAL THINKING CASE STUDY

1. Mrs. J.'s knowledge base should be assessed. Mrs. J. needs to avoid concentrated sweets and eat 4 to 6 small balanced meals to maintain an adequate blood sugar. Symptoms of hypo- and hyperglycemia should be reviewed. She should also be taught how to handle her diabetes when she becomes ill.

2. Mrs. J. should be checking her blood glucose levels regularly, recording them, and sharing them with her physician so that he can adjust her insulin. Mrs. J. is experiencing hypoglycemia during the night; therefore her evening dose of NPH may need to be decreased. She may also need to increase her caloric intake at night. You should also find out if Mrs. J. is exercising in the evening.

3. Ask if he can get Mrs. J. to drink. If she can, he should use a high carbohydrate drink. If she cannot drink and there is glucagon in the house, he should administer it. If neither of the aforementioned things are possible, he should immediately bring her to the emergency room.

4. NPH peaks in approximately 8 hours. If Mrs. P. is taking NPH insulin at supper time (6 p.m.), it peaks at approximately 2 a.m. By changing NPH to 10 p.m., it will be peaking at 6 a.m.

28
Estrogens, Progestins, and Oral Contraceptives

MAJOR TOPICS

Functions of endogenous estrogens
Drug formulations of estrogens and progestins

DRUG LIST

Estrogens (Premarin, Estrace, Estraderm)
Medroxyprogesterone (Provera)

OBJECTIVES

1. Discuss effects of endogenous estrogens and progestins.
2. Describe advantages and disadvantages of
   postmenopausal hormone replacement therapy (HRT).
3. Describe adverse effects associated with estrogens,
   progestins, and oral contraceptives.

TEACHING STRATEGIES

Classroom

1. If oral contraceptives are included in a maternal-
   child nursing course, the instructor may wish to
   omit or minimize discussion in the pharmacology class. Two of the most commonly used preparations are Ortho-Novum 7/7/7 and Triphasil.

2. Assign two groups of students to debate the issue
   of hormone replacement therapy (HRT) for
   menopausal women.

3. Discuss advantages and disadvantages of HRT.

4. Discuss the Critical Thinking Case Study related
   to oral contraceptives (SG, p. 104).

Clinical Laboratory

1. For clients receiving estrogen or progesterone,
   have students assess age, reason for use, and current or potential adverse effects.

2. For clients receiving an oral contraceptive, have
   students assess for risk factors and for signs and
   symptoms of deep vein thrombosis.

3. For a 40-year-old woman with a recent hysterec-
   tomy and bilateral oophorectomy (surgical
   menopause), discuss teaching needs in relation to
   estrogen replacement therapy.

TESTBANK QUESTIONS

1. Birth control pill users are at increased risk for:
   a. cancer.
   b. hyponatremia.
   *c. thrombophlebitis.
   d. psychosis.

2. Which of the following statements by your
client, who was started on estrogen for prostatic
cancer, leads you to believe that he has understood the teaching that you have done?
   a. "Hair loss is common, so I will use Rogaine."
   b. "I may experience impotence, which will be
      permanent."
   c. "I will take this medication for the rest of my
      life."
   *d. "I will not become alarmed if my breasts
      enlarge."

3. Mrs. K., a 35-year-old mother of 2, has a history
   of smoking and chronic fatigue. She is also on a
   low-sodium diet for renal insufficiency. Which
   factors in Mrs. K.'s history would contraindicate
   the use of birth control pills?
   a. Chronic fatigue
   b. Age
   *c. Smoking
   d. Renal insufficiency

4. Conjugated estrogens (Premarin) are administered to prevent:
   a. endometriosis.
   *b. dysfunctional uterine bleeding.
   c. osteoporosis.
   d. uterine cancer.

5. The following medication may be administered
   to men with prostatic cancer:
   a. Estropipate (Ogen)
   b. Medroxyprogesterone acetate (Provera)
   *c. Ethinyl estradiol (Estinyl)
   d. Quinestrol (Estrovis)

6. The following medications, when administered
   concurrently with oral contraceptives, will
   decrease their effect:
   *a. Antimicrobial drugs
   b. Antihypertensive drugs
   c. Anti-inflammatory drugs
   d. Anticholinergic drugs

7. Women taking estrogen need to be assessed for
   the following adverse effect:
   a. Weight loss
   *b. Hyperglycemia
   c. Gynecomastia
   d. Dysrhythmias

8. Estrogen replacement is given to postmenopausal
   women to prevent:
   a. stroke.
   *b. osteoporosis.
   c. premature aging.
   d. sexual disinterest.

CRITICAL THINKING CASE STUDY

1. Factors that would preclude the use of birth control pills include pregnancy, thromboembolic
   disorders (they increase hepatic production of
   clotting factors), cancer (they can stimulate
   tumor growth), hypertension (they increase

angiotension and sodium and water retention), and women over 35 who smoke (they cause increased platelet aggregation).

2. Before drug therapy is started, the client needs a comprehensive physical examination, including measurements of blood pressure, cholesterol, and triglyceride levels.

3. Persons can experience weight gain and acne from taking oral contraceptives. Mrs. G. needs to continue to take the medication and make an appointment with her physician. He may change her medication, which could alleviate the problem.

29
Androgens and Anabolic Steroids

MAJOR TOPICS

Functions of androgens
Abuse of anabolic steroids

DRUG LIST

Danazol (Danocrine)
Testosterone

OBJECTIVES

1. Discuss effects of endogenous androgens.
2. Discuss uses and effects of exogenous androgens and anabolic steroids.
3. Discuss the rationale for using danazol to treat women with endometriosis or fibrocystic breast disease.
4. Describe potential consequences of abusing anabolic steroids.

TEACHING STRATEGIES

Classroom

1. Because these drugs are infrequently given in most clinical settings, the instructor may choose to omit them or minimize class time.

2. Review (or have students review independently) physiologic effects of endogenous androgens.

3. Discuss effects of androgens on women and children.

4. Ask students if they know other students who take anabolic steroids. If so, ask them to share their observations about appearances and behaviors of the drug-takers and their thoughts about adverse effects of the drugs.

5. Discuss the Critical Thinking Case Study (SG, p. 107).

Clinical Laboratory

1. For women receiving danazol, have students assess for masculinizing effects.

2. For children receiving testosterone, ask students to assess the parents' knowledge about and willingness to comply with the recommendation for x-rays every 6 months.

TESTBANK QUESTIONS

1. When anabolic steroids are administered the individual may experience:
   a. increased pulse rate.
   b. decreased white blood cell count.
   *c. increased serum calcium levels.
   d. decreased bone growth.

2. An insulin dependent diabetic is started on testosterone for cryptorchidism. Which of the following statements by J. leads you to believe that he has understood the teaching you have done?
   a. "My dose of insulin will not need to be adjusted."
   *b. "My insulin dose may need to be decreased."
   c. "My dose of insulin may need to be increased."
   d. "My insulin will be discontinued while I am taking this drug."

3. An expected outcome of the administration of fluoxymesterone (Halotestin) for hypogonadism is:
   *a. growth of sexual organs.
   b. decreased skin thickness.
   c. increased protein metabolism.
   d. retention of potassium.

4. Long-term use of high doses of anabolic steroids can cause the following adverse effect:
   a. Impotence
   b. Immobility of joints
   c. Obesity
   *d. Hypertension

5. A change that can occur in adult females with the use of androgens is:
   a. enlargement of breasts.
   b. hair loss.
   *c. suppression of menstruation.
   d. increase in height.

6. An expected outcome when nandrolone phenpropionate (Durabolin) is administered is an increase in:
   a. folic acid levels.
   *b. red blood cell count.
   c. platelet count.
   d. vitamin B_{12} levels.

7. An expected outcome when androgens are administered for breast cancer is an increase in:
   a. sexual desire.
   *b. feeling of well being.
   c. muscle strength.
   d. lung capacity.

8. Androgens potentiate the effect of insulin. There-fore the dose may need to be:
   a. increased significantly.
   b. adjusted daily.
   *c. decreased.
   d. eliminated.

9. Women who are receiving androgen treatment for breast cancer need to have the following elec-trolyte evaluated regularly:
   a. Sodium
   b. Potassium
   c. Chloride
   *d. Calcium

CRITICAL THINKING CASE STUDY

1. As teenagers, you believe that there are benefits to steroid use. Yes, you can get some increase in muscle mass, strength, and weight. You also need to be aware of the negative effects of steroid use that far outweigh the positive effects. Large doses of steroids cause a variety of liver disorders that can lead to hemorrhage or liver failure. Behav-ioral changes have been documented, including aggressiveness, hostility, and combativeness. Dependence can occur, which is characterized by preoccupation with drug use, inability to stop taking the drugs, and withdrawal symptoms. Large doses of steroids can result in testicular atrophy, low sperm counts, and impotence in men, and there is an increased risk of cardiovas-cular disease. Severe acne can also occur.

2. Physical changes indicative of steroid use that the nurse could be assessing for include:
   a. deepened voice.
   b. increased muscle mass (the nurse could mea-sure muscle mass).
   c. weight gain (the nurse could check students' weights and also vital signs for a possible increase in blood pressure due to fluid reten-tion).
   d. increased serum cholesterol levels (the nurse could monitor serum cholesterol levels).

V

NUTRIENTS, FLUIDS, AND ELECTROLYTES

30
Nutritional Products, Anorexiants, and Digestants

MAJOR TOPICS

Characteristics, functions, requirements, and food sources
    of water, carbohydrates, proteins, and fats
Fluid disorders
Enteral and parenteral nutrition
Overnutrition (Obesity)
Undernutrition

PRODUCT AND DRUG LIST

Ensure
Fenfluramine (Pondimin)
Osmolite
Pancrelipase (Viokase)
Phentermine (Fastin, Ionamin)
Phenylpropanolamine (Accutrim, Dexatrim)
Pulmocare
TraumaCal

OBJECTIVES

1. Discuss the importance of water, carbohydrates, proteins, and fats in maintaining health.
2. Identify clients at risk of developing fluid disorders.
3. Identify clients at risk of developing undernutrition.
4. Discuss nutrients needed to promote tissue healing and recovery from illness.
5. Discuss common disorders and drugs that interfere with nutrition.
6. Describe nursing interventions to maintain fluid balance.
7. Describe nursing interventions to increase calorie-protein intake in undernourished clients.
8. Review health consequences of obesity.
9. Discuss nursing interventions to assist obese clients in weight management.

TEACHING STRATEGIES

Classroom

1. Differentiate nursing and dietary responsibilities in nutritional assessment and teaching.

2. Ask students to compare enteral and parenteral nutrition in terms of convenience to the client, efficacy, and adverse effects.
3. Discuss review and application exercise 9 (text, p. 390).
4. Discuss nutritional support of clients with cancer.
5. Assign the Critical Thinking Case Study (SG, p. 113) as a homework assignment to be turned in.
6. Discuss review and application exercise 10 (text, p. 391).

Clinical Laboratory

1. Have students assess all assigned clients for risks of fluid and nutritional imbalances.
2. Have the clinical group analyze weight and height of selected clients to assist in determining nutritional status.
3. Have the clinical group evaluate drugs ordered for a client in terms of potential interference with fluid and nutritional needs.
4. For a client receiving intravenous fluids, have students analyze the fluids and nutrients provided per 24 hours and compare them with recommended amounts.
5. For a client receiving central or peripheral parenteral nutrition, interview the client and demonstrate the apparatus to students.
6. For a client receiving a supplementary enteral feeding, have students analyze the amount taken in relation to the amount needed.

TESTBANK QUESTIONS

1. Milk-based formulas are:
    *a. used for clients with a functioning gastrointestinal tract.
    b. low in protein and high in carbohydrates.
    c. high in vitamins and minerals but low in carbohydrates.
    d. used in clients with lactose intolerance.

2. Which of the following statements is true regarding commercial formulas used for enteral feedings?
   a. Most formulas provide 5 calories per ml when administered at full strength.
   b. The protein content is 50% of the total calories.
   c. Formulas that have a low osmolarity tend to cause constipation.
   *d. Fats increase the calories without increasing osmolarity.

3. Your client is receiving half a can of Ensure and 120 ml of H_2O q4h. How many calories will she receive per day?
   *a. 760 calories
   b. 805 calories
   c. 960 calories
   d. 1540 calories

4. During the initial administration of a fat emulsion, the nurse should:
   a. administer the emulsion at a rate of 5 ml/minute for the first hour.
   *b. observe for signs of a fat embolus.
   c. use an in-line filter for IV administration.
   d. observe for renal shutdown.

5. When observing a client receiving enteral feedings, the nurse should be aware that:
   *a. formulas with high osmolarity can cause diarrhea and dehydration.
   b. hyperosmolar-induced edema can occur with tube feedings that have a high fat content.
   c. if Mrs. G. has a food allergy, she will still be able to tolerate enteral feeding without a reaction.
   d. a red macular rash may be a precursor of hyperosmolar shock.

6. Mr. P. experiences respiratory distress during the administration of a continuous tube feeding. After stopping the feeding you should first:
   a. assess bowel sound to determine if he has a paralytic ileus.
   *b. assess breath sounds to determine if he has aspirated.
   c. nasally or tracheally suction Mr. P.
   d. palpate his abdomen and aspirate the stomach contents.

7. A nursing action for a client receiving TPN would be to:
   a. change the catheter dressing daily.
   *b. start the solution rate slowly at 50 ml/hour.
   c. change the TPN solution every 48 hours.
   d. hang Lactated Ringer's if the TPN is interrupted.

8. An assessment that should be performed daily for a client receiving TPN is:
   a. abdominal girth.
   b. serum calcium levels.
   c. ECG.
   *d. weight.

9. The following lab data should be assessed routinely for a client receiving parenteral nutrition:
   a. T_3 and T_4 levels
   b. Urine amylase
   *c. Serum glucose
   d. Creatinine clearance

10. Which of the following statements by Mr. C.'s daughter, who will care for him at home, leads you to believe that she has understood your teaching regarding tube feedings? "I will:
    a. store the unopened cans in the refrigerator."
    b. stop the feedings if he has more than 2 stools per day."
    *c. place him in a sitting position for his feedings."
    d. give no more than 100 cc/hour."

11. A client with burns over 50% of his body receives Trauma Cal because:
    *a. it is a high protein formula with easily assimilated amino acids.
    b. its metabolism produces less carbon dioxide.
    c. it requires no digestion and leaves no fecal residue.
    d. it supplies large amounts of protein but few carbohydrates and no fat.

12. Which of the following statements by the mother of a child with cystic fibrosis leads you to believe that she understands how pancrelipase (Viokase) is to be administered at home?
    *a. "I will mix the powder with his food at each meal."
    b. "I will administer the medication via enema at bedtime."
    c. "I will administer the medication via nebulizer a.c. and h.s."
    d. "I will give the medication on an empty stomach."

13. Which of the following symptoms of a protein deficit would you expect to see initially in a child with malnutrition?
    a. Increased hemoglobin
    b. Alkalosis
    *c. Dry skin
    d. Tachycardia

14. Modular formulas such as Polycose:
    a. are used for persons whose GI tracts are not functioning.
    b. provide complete nutrition.
    *c. provide single nutrients used to supplement oral intake.
    d. contain lactose and may cause diarrhea.

15. Hydrolyzed formulas are used for clients who:
    a. need a high fat formula.
    *b. have an impaired GI tract.
    c. need increased fiber.
    d. require soy as their protein source.

16. The following formula has a high fat content and minimizes CO_2 production:
    a. Amin-Aid
    b. Hepatic-Aid
    c. Immun-Aid
    *d. Pulmocare

17. Prior to administering tube feedings, the nurse should check the client's:
    a. vital signs.
    *b. residual stomach contents.
    c. breath sounds.
    d. neurologic status.

18. Trauma Cal is used because it:
    *a. promotes wound healing.
    b. prevents cramping and diarrhea.
    c. improves bowel function.
    d. eliminates peripheral edema.

19. A lab test to evaluate the effectiveness of enteral feedings is:
    *a. total proteins.
    b. blood urea nitrogen.
    c. serum glucose.
    d. serum sodium.

20. Symptoms of hypomagnesemia that a client receiving TPN can exhibit include:
    a. lethargy, abdominal cramps, and sweating.
    *b. tremors, tachycardia, and confusion.
    c. ascites and distended neck veins.
    d. peripheral edema and neuropathy.

CRITICAL THINKING CASE STUDY

1. Pulmocare was chosen because it is the supplemental feeding of choice for clients with chronic obstructive pulmonary disease (COPD). Because of the impaired breathing, these clients have difficulty eliminating sufficient quantities of CO_2, a waste product of carbohydrate metabolism. When CO_2 accumulates in the body, it may produce respiratory acidosis and eventually respiratory failure. Pulmocare contains more fat (55%) and less carbohydrates (28%) than most other formulas. Consequently, its metabolism produces less CO_2. It contains 1.5 cal/ml. Mr. J. is to receive 2000 ml of Pulmocare per 24 hours. Therefore, he will receive 83 ml/hr:

$$\frac{2,000 \text{ ml}}{24} = 83.3 \ (83) \text{ ml/hr.}$$

    His caloric intake will be 3000 cal/day: 2000 ml $\times$ 1.5 cal. The 3000 cal/day are sufficient to maintain his present weight.

2. The nurse should be assessing for diarrhea, fluid volume deficit, hypernatremia, and aspiration of the formula into the lungs.

3. TPN is expensive, irritating to the vessels, and can cause hyperglycemia and septicemia. It is useful in individuals who do not have a functioning GI tract. Mr. J. was probably started on enteral feedings because they are inexpensive and convenient (a person can easily be transferred home or to a long-term care facility).

4. Aspiration is a common problem associated with tube feedings. It can be prevented by proper positioning, checking for tube placement, checking residual stomach content, and giving feedings slowly. Dehydration is another problem. Unless otherwise indicated, all persons receiving tube feedings should receive 1500–3000 ml of water daily.

5. Diarrhea is usually attributed to the hypertonicity of the preparations. Diarrhea can be prevented by starting with small amounts of dilute solutions and gradually increasing to full strength. The nurse should assess Mr. J.'s skin and his lab values and notify the physician that Mr. J. is having diarrhea. The physician may decrease the strength of the tube feeding or order an antidiarrheal.

31
Vitamins

MAJOR TOPICS

Types, functions, requirements, and food sources of vitamins

MULTIVITAMIN PREPARATIONS

Stuart's prenatal vitamins
Theragran
ViDaylin

OBJECTIVES

1. Review functions and food sources of essential vitamins.
2. Differentiate between maintenance and therapeutic doses of vitamins.
3. Identify clients at risk of developing vitamin deficiency or overdose.
4. Delineate circumstances in which therapeutic vitamins are likely to be needed.
5. Describe adverse effects associated with overdose of fat-soluble and selected water-soluble vitamins.
6. Discuss the rationale for administering vitamin K to newborns.

TEACHING STRATEGIES

Classroom

1. Students who have had a nutrition class may need only to review basic content and some discussion of vitamins-as-drugs.

2. Discuss use of RDAs in personal life to promote health and well-being.

3. Review ways to cook and store food to retain vitamin content.

4. Discuss the pros and cons of taking vitamin supplements.

5. Have small groups of students analyze OTC multivitamin preparations (e.g., adult and children's multivitamins and a prenatal vitamin) in relation to the RDAs for the intended population.

6. Discuss or assign to small groups the Critical Thinking Case Study (SG, p. 116).

Clinical Laboratory

1. Have students assess assigned clients for actual or potential vitamin deficiency.

2. Ask students to teach clients ways to increase their dietary intake of vitamins.

3. Encourage students to teach clients (and others) to avoid megadoses of any vitamins, whenever an opportunity arises.

TESTBANK QUESTIONS

1. A client who smokes cigarettes is likely to experience a deficiency in:
   a. vitamin A.
   b. vitamin B_{12}.
   *c. vitamin C.
   d. vitamin D.

2. Antibiotics administered in conjunction with vitamin K may:
   a. cause bleeding due to increased APT times.
   *b. decrease its effects.
   c. increase intestinal absorption of vitamin K.
   d. alter liver function studies.

3. Your client is to receive 26,250 units of vitamin A per day for 10 days. If the medication comes in a vial labeled 1 cc = 35,000 units, how many milliliters will you administer?
   a. 0.55 ml
   b. 0.65 ml
   *c. 0.75 ml
   d. 0.85 ml

4. Exposure to the sun is necessary to provide adequate amounts of vitamin:
   a. A.
   b. B_{12}.
   c. K.
   *d. D.

5. Vitamin D absorption is impaired by:
   a. obesity.
   *b. mineral oil.
   c. high carbohydrate diet.
   d. decreased protein intake.

6. Concurrent administration of pyridoxine (vitamin B_6) interferes with:
   a. warfarin (Coumadin).
   b. phenytoin (Dilantin).
   *c. levodopa (Larodopa).
   d. diazepam (Valium).

7. The following test is used to diagnose pernicious anemia:
   *a. Schilling test
   b. Agglutination test
   c. Dick test
   d. CBC

8. Chronic alcoholics often have the following vitamin deficiencies:
   a. Pyridoxine (B_6) and vitamin E
   b. Ascorbic acid (C) and riboflavin (B_2)
   *c. Thiamine (B_1) and folic acid
   d. Cyanocobalamin (B_{12}) and vitamin A

9. Foods high in vitamin K should be avoided if a client is taking:
   *a. warfarin (Coumadin).
   b. vitamin B_{12}.
   c. phenobarbital.
   d. furosemide (Lasix).

10. An expected outcome after the administration of vitamin B_{12} is:
    a. decreased bleeding.
    *b. increased energy level.
    c. decreased heart rate.
    d. improved vision.

CRITICAL THINKING CASE STUDY

1. This would include a complete assessment, as well as blood work, because all body systems can be affected by malnutrition.

2. Niacin is essential for glycolysis, fat synthesis, and fat metabolism; when niacin is lacking, the individual can develop pellagra. Thiamine is essential for energy production. A mild deficiency will cause fatigue, anorexia, growth retardation, depression, and irritability. A severe deficiency causes peripheral neuritis, personality disturbances, and heart failure. Folic acid is essential for metabolism, normal red blood cells, and growth. Megaloblastic anemia, impaired growth in children, and GI problems can result from a folic acid deficiency. Vitamins are administered parenterally if severe GI malabsorption exists or the disease is severe.

3. After discussing the rationale for administering the medication with Mr. B., if he still refuses the injections, contact his physician. The medication can be given orally.

32
Minerals and Electrolytes

MAJOR TOPICS

Minerals as nutrients
Deficiency and excess states of sodium, potassium, and magnesium
Drugs used in treatment of deficiency and excess states

DRUG LIST

Deferoxamine (Desferal)
Ferrous sulfate (FeSO$_4$)
Magnesium sulfate (MgSO$_4$)
Potassium chloride (KC1) (K-Dur, Klor-Con)
Sodium polystyrene sulfonate (Kayexalate)
Succinimide (Chemet)

OBJECTIVES

1. Discuss functions and food sources of major minerals.
2. Identify clients at risk of developing selected mineral and electrolyte imbalances.
3. Describe signs, symptoms, and treatments of sodium, potassium, and magnesium imbalances.
4. Describe signs, symptoms, and treatment of iron deficiency anemia.
5. Discuss the chelating agents used to remove excessive copper, iron, and lead from tissues.
6. Apply nursing process skills to prevent, recognize, or treat mineral/electrolyte imbalances.

TEACHING STRATEGIES

Classroom

1. Compare potassium content in selected food sources, salt substitutes, and prescription KC1 preparations.

2. Ask students about their experiences with clients who were receiving KC1.

3. Ask students about personal intake of iron and whether they think they receive an adequate amount.

4. Assign the Critical Thinking Case Study (SG, p. 119) for small group discussion, then discuss as a class.

Clinical Laboratory

1. Have students assess assigned clients in relation to electrolyte balance, including usual eating habits and laboratory reports of serum sodium, potassium, and magnesium.

2. For clients receiving a potassium-losing diuretic, have students check serum K before giving.

3. Have students assess assigned clients for iron deficiency anemia, including serum iron and iron binding capacity if available.

4. In a home care setting, assess the environment for risk factors related to overdoses of iron, lead, potassium, and other metals.

TESTBANK QUESTIONS

1. The drug used to treat metabolic acidosis is:
   a. ammonium chloride.
   b. deferoxamine (Desferal).
   *c. sodium bicarbonate.
   d. magnesium sulfate.

2. Which of the following instructions is important to include in discharge teaching for a client taking an iron preparation? "This medication:
   *a. may turn your stools dark green or black."
   b. will cause you to have diarrhea."
   c. should be taken with an antacid."
   d. should not be taken with fruit juice."

3. The following electrolyte solution should never be administered as an undiluted bolus because it can cause fatal dysrhythmias:
   a. Sodium chloride
   *b. Potassium chloride
   c. Magnesium sulfate
   d. Sodium bicarbonate

4. The most abundant cation in the intracellular compartment is:
   a. sodium.
   b. chloride.
   *c. potassium.
   d. magnesium.

5. Elevated serum sodium levels will decrease the effectiveness of:
   a. digoxin (Lanoxin).
   *b. lithium carbonate (Eskalith).
   c. furosemide (Lasix).
   d. propranolol (Inderal).

6. A client is admitted with muscle weakness, lethargy, and hypotension. The electrolyte imbalance associated with these symptoms is:
   *a. hypermagnesemia.
   b. hypophosphatemia.
   c. hyperkalemia.
   d. hypochloremia.

7. After 2 months on total parenteral nutrition, your client exhibits irritability, tetany, and tremors. The electrolyte imbalance associated with these symptoms is:
   a. hypophosphatemia.
   b. hyperkalemia.
   c. hypercalcemia.
   *d. hypomagnesemia.

8. A copper deficiency can cause:
   *a. anemia.
   b. excessive perspiration.
   c. impaired reproduction.
   d. hyperglycemia.

9. The following element is obtained from ingestion of animal proteins:
   a. Chromium
   b. Iodine
   *c. Zinc
   d. Potassium

10. High intake of liver, shellfish, nuts, and dried fruits can result in elevated levels of:
    *a. copper.
    b. cobalt.
    c. selenium.
    d. iodine.

CRITICAL THINKING CASE STUDY

1. A client in renal failure requires a complete assessment because this disease effects every body system. Besides assessing orientation, vital signs, I and O, weight, and presence of edema, the nurse must also monitor the client's cardiac status.

2. Dysrhythmias can occur with hyperkalemia, acidosis, alkalosis, and hypocalcemia. As Mr. B. is being treated for acidosis, the nurse must monitor the electrolyte changes carefully. Sodium bicarbonate is used to treat acidosis but can produce alkalosis, and alkalosis causes hypocalcemia. Acidosis is associated with hyperkalemia.

3. Your serum potassium levels are still very high. We must bring them down so that you will not have any heart problems. The medication that we are giving you acts in your colon, therefore if we give it rectally it will work more rapidly.

VI
DRUGS USED TO TREAT INFECTIONS

33
General Characteristics of Antimicrobial Drugs

MAJOR TOPICS

Host defense mechanisms
Common pathogenic microorganisms
Antibiotic-resistant microorganisms
Use of drugs in children and elderly adults
Use of drugs with renal insufficiency and liver disease

OBJECTIVES

1. Identify populations who are at increased risk of developing infections.
2. Discuss common pathogens and methods of infection control.
3. Assess clients for local and systemic signs of infection.
4. Discuss common and potentially serious adverse effects of antimicrobial drugs.
5. Identify clients at increased risk of adverse drug reactions.
6. Discuss ways to increase benefits and decrease hazards of antimicrobial drug therapy.
7. Discuss ways to minimize emergence of drug-resistant microorganisms.
8. State appropriate nursing implications for a client receiving an antimicrobial drug.
9. Discuss important elements of using antimicrobial drugs in children and older adults.

TEACHING STRATEGIES

Classroom

1. Lecture/discussion using the objectives as an outline.
2. Assign students to write definitions for any new or unclear terms.
3. Discuss risk factors for developing an infection.
4. Discuss circumstances in which a person is likely to develop an infection with antibiotic-resistant microorganisms.
5. Discuss or have students write answers to the review and application exercises (text, p. 452).
6. Assign two groups of students to debate the issue of antibiotic use (e.g., Resolved: Overuse and inappropriate use of antibiotics endangers the public health).

7. Assign small groups to prepare a general teaching plan about an antibiotic.
8. Discuss ways nurses can promote rational use of antimicrobial drugs.
9. Ask a pharmacist or infection control nurse to speak to the class about local patterns of microbial resistance to antibiotics, difficulties in treating infections caused by antibiotic-resistant microorganisms, and CDC or personal recommendations for preventing emergence of drug-resistant microorganisms.
10. Assign students to obtain, read, and summarize (verbally for the class and written for the instructor) a journal article related to some aspect of preventing, recognizing, or managing infectious disease. The instructor may wish to list the names of some journals that are available and likely to contain appropriate articles.

Clinical Laboratory

1. For clients with increased risk of developing infection, have students plan and implement interventions to decrease the risk.
2. For clients with infections, ask students to verbalize assessment data, give at least one nursing diagnosis, and state interventions to protect themselves and others in the environment.
3. For clients receiving an antimicrobial drug, have students check culture and susceptibility reports if available, look up the specific drug, and evaluate whether the ordered drug is appropriate for the particular client.
4. For clients receiving an antimicrobial drug, have students obtain and individualize instructions for use.
5. Have students discuss the importance of taking antimicrobial drugs as prescribed.
6. In hospital settings with an infection control nurse, ask the nurse to conduct a postclinical conference about nurses' roles and responsibilities in infection control.

TESTBANK QUESTIONS

1. Routine ingestion of the following medication predisposes persons to infection:
   a. Insulin
   *b. Corticosteroids
   c. Beta-adrenergic blockers
   d. Anti-infectives

2. A nosocomial infection is:
   *a. acquired in the hospital.
   b. caused by the use of antibiotics.
   c. spread by contaminated food.
   d. contracted only by persons who are immuno-suppressed.

3. Tetracyclines are most effective if taken:
   a. before bed time.
   *b. on an empty stomach.
   c. with 12 ounces of water.
   d. with a full glass of milk.

4. Subjective symptoms of infection include:
   a. tachycardia.
   b. fever.
   c. elevated WBC.
   *d. lethargy.

5. The following electrolyte may elevate in persons receiving penicillin therapy:
   a. Sodium
   b. Chloride
   c. Calcium
   *d. Potassium

6. A client receiving intravenous aminoglycoside therapy should be assessed daily for:
   a. hematuria.
   *b. hearing loss.
   c. angina.
   d. dysrhythmias.

7. The following lab study should be monitored daily for a client receiving parenteral aminogly-cosides:
   a. Serum albumin
   b. Serum calcium
   *c. Serum creatinine
   d. Urine osmolarity

8. A client with a sensitivity to which of the following drugs may also have a sensitivity to cefazolin (Ancef)?
   *a. Penicillin
   b. Tetracycline
   c. Sulfa
   d. Streptomycin

9. A diabetic taking oral agents may become hypo-glycemic if placed on:
   a. tetracyclines.
   b. penicillins.
   *c. sulfonamides.
   d. aminoglycosides.

10. Your client has pneumonia, and his physician has ordered a second antibiotic. Your client has a triple lumen catheter in place. You should:
    a. administer both medications simultaneously.
    b. start the second antibiotic as soon as the first is finished.
    *c. monitor the client's WBC daily.
    d. obtain a sputum specimen after 2 doses of the medication have been given.

34
Beta-Lactam Antibacterials: Penicillins, Cephalosporins, and Others

MAJOR TOPICS

Characteristics of beta lactam antibacterial drugs
Beta lactamase enzymes
Evolution of subgroups of penicillins
Beta lactamase inhibitor drugs
Comparison of cephalosporins to penicillins
Similarities and differences between "generations" of cephalosporins

DRUG LIST
Penicillins

Amoxicillin (Amoxil, Trimox)
Amoxicillin/clavulanate (Augmentin)
Ampicillin (Principen)
Ampicillin/sulbactam (Unasyn)
Dicloxacillin (Dynapen)
Piperacillin (Pipracil)
Piperacillin/tazobactam (Zosyn)
Ticarcillin (Ticar)
Ticarcillin/clavulanate (Timentin)
Penicillin G
Penicillin V (Veetids)

Cephalosporins

Cefaclor (Ceclor)
Cefadroxil (Duricef)
Cefazolin (Kefzol, Ancef)
Cefixime (Suprax)
Cefoperazone (Cefobid)
Cefprozil (Cefzil)
Ceftazidime (Fortaz)
Ceftriaxone (Rocephin)
Cefuroxime (Ceftin)

Others

Aztreonam (Azactam)
Imipenem/cilastatin (Primaxin)
Meropenem (Merrem)

OBJECTIVES

1. Describe general characteristics of beta lactam antibiotics.
2. Discuss penicillins in relation to effectiveness, safety, spectrum of antimicrobial activity, mechanism of action, indications for use, administration, observation of client response, and teaching of clients.
3. Differentiate among extended-spectrum penicillins.
4. Question clients about allergies prior to the initial dose of a penicillin.
5. Describe characteristics of beta lactamase inhibitor drugs.
6. State the rationale for combining a penicillin and a beta lactamase inhibitor drug.
7. Discuss similarities and differences between cephalosporins and penicillins.
8. Differentiate among the four generations of cephalosporins in relation to antimicrobial spectrum, indications for use, and adverse effects.
9. Apply principles of using beta lactam antimicrobials in selected client situations.

TEACHING STRATEGIES

Classroom

1. Show a transparency of the four types of beta lactam drugs (IM, p. 143).
2. Show a transparency of the beta lactam chemical structure (IM, p. 143).
3. Show a transparency of the listed penicillins, and remind students that generic names ending in "cillin" are penicillins.
4. Show a transparency of each "generation" of cephalosporins (IM, p. 144–146). Because there are so many of these drugs, the instructor may wish to determine the ones most often used in local agencies and communities.
5. Note that the generic names of all cephalosporins except loracarbef and moxalactam (which are synthetic drugs) begin with "cef" or "ceph."
6. Discuss the role of cephalosporins in surgical chemoprophylaxis.
7. Discuss the review and application exercises (text, p. 471).
8. Assign small groups to prepare a general teaching plan for oral penicillins, then compare their plan with a drug reference on an individual penicillin (amoxicillin is the most commonly used for ambulatory clients).
9. Assign pairs to list the main client teaching points for a randomly selected oral or parenteral cephalosporin. Then, have two pairs (both with an oral drug or a parenteral drug) compare their plans and indicate any differences. Ask that written work be signed by pair members and turned in.
10. Assign students to write answers to the Critical Thinking Case Study (SG, p. 127) and turn in for a grade.

Clinical Laboratory

1. For a group of clients, have students identify those who are receiving a penicillin (or the instructor can identify from medication records) and discuss reasons for use and drug effects in particular clients.
2. For clients who are receiving a penicillin, ask students to identify the group or subgroup, the dose and route of administration, and describe a rationale for using the drug, the dose, and the route for a particular client.
3. For clients receiving a cephalosporin, have students review culture and susceptibility reports, the location of the infection or surgical procedure, and the specific drug; then, have students evaluate the appropriateness of the drug for the particular client.
4. For clients receiving an IV penicillin or cephalosporin, discuss how the drug is provided and IV fluids with which the drug is mixed.
5. For clients receiving a beta lactam drug, ask students to assess for adverse effects and verbally report findings in a postclinical conference.
6. For a client newly started on an oral penicillin or cephalosporin, obtain an instruction sheet and discuss ways to individualize the instructions.

TESTBANK QUESTIONS

1. *Candida* infections, seen as a result of broad spectrum antibiotic use, can cause:
   a. nausea, vomiting, and diarrhea.
   b. a macular rash.
   *c. vaginal discharge and sore mouth.
   d. high-grade fever and seizures.

2. The excretion of penicillin can be prolonged by administration of:
   a. allopurinol (Zyloprim).
   b. furosemide (Lasix).
   c. ascorbic acid (vitamin C).
   *d. probenecid (Benemid).

3. A serious reaction related to the use of penicillin is:
   a. neurotoxicity.
   *b. anaphylactic reaction.
   c. renal failure.
   d. leukopenia.

4. Penicillins work by inhibiting:
   a. protein synthesis.
   b. DNA replication.
   *c. cell wall synthesis.
   d. leukocytes.

5. Augmentin:
   a. is administered to individuals who have built up a tolerance to penicillin.
   *b. combines a penicillin derivative with a beta lactamase inhibitor.
   c. is effective when all other antibiotics have been ineffective.
   d. is used in children because it has no adverse effects.

6. The concurrent administration of the following antibiotic with birth control pills decreases their effectiveness:
   a. Methicillin
   *b. Ampicillin
   c. Ticarcillin
   d. Carbenicillin

7. When administering cephalosporins, you need to assess the client for:
   a. ototoxicity.
   b. phototoxicity.
   *c. nephrotoxicity.
   d. hepatotoxicity.

8. Compared to amoxicillin, ampicillin causes a higher incidence of:
   *a. nausea and diarrhea.
   b. photosensitivity.
   c. anaphylactic reactions.
   d. gastrointestinal bleeding.

9. The most accurate way to identify nephrotoxicity in a client receiving a cephalosporin is to assess:
   a. urinary output.
   b. weight and blood pressure.
   *c. serum creatinine levels.
   d. blood urea nitrogen levels.

10. The following cephalosporin can cause hypoprothrombinemia:
    *a. Cefoperazone (Cefobid)
    b. Cefotaxime (Claforan)
    c. Ceftazidime (Fortaz)
    d. Ceftriaxone (Rocephin)

CRITICAL THINKING CASE STUDY

1. Ampicillin is a broad spectrum, semisynthetic penicillin that is bactericidal for several types of gram-positive and gram-negative bacteria. It is effective in treating Shigella infections.

2. The route of choice depends on the seriousness of the infection. Normally this type of infection would be treated with oral antibiotics, but Mr. B. is an insulin dependent diabetic. An infectious process can elevate his blood sugar. Since Mr. B. is also dehydrated, intravenous therapy is appropriate in his case.

3. Perform a complete assessment, including vital signs and respiratory assessment. A rash is a hypersensitivity reaction and his physician should be notified.

35
Aminoglycosides and Fluoroquinolones

MAJOR TOPICS

Types of infections for which aminoglycosides are used
Comparison with beta lactam antibiotics
Fluoroquinolones

DRUG LIST

Amikacin (Amikin)
Ciprofloxacin (Cipro)
Enoxacin (Penetrex)
Gentamicin (Garamycin)
Lomefloxacin (Maxaquin)
Ofloxacin (Floxin)
Tobramycin (Nebcin)

OBJECTIVES

1. Describe characteristics of aminoglycosides in relation to effectiveness, safety, spectrum of antimicrobial activity, indications for use, administration, and observation of client responses.
2. Discuss factors influencing selection and dosage of aminoglycosides.
3. State the rationale for the increasing use of single daily doses rather than multiple daily doses.
4. Discuss the importance of serum drug levels during aminoglycoside therapy.
5. Describe measures to prevent or minimize nephrotoxicity and ototoxicity with aminoglycosides.
6. Describe characteristics, uses, adverse effects, and nursing process implications of fluoroquinolones.
7. Apply principles of using aminoglycosides and fluoroquinolones in selected client situations.

TEACHING STRATEGIES

Classroom

1. Lecture/discussion about uses and effects of aminoglycosides, according to objectives.
2. Show a transparency of aminoglycoside drug names (IM, p. 147).
3. Emphasize gentamicin as the most commonly used aminoglycoside.
4. Discuss review and application exercises 1–10 (text, p. 481).
5. Discuss the Critical Thinking Case Study (SG, p. 129) as a class.
6. Lecture/discussion about uses and effects of fluoroquinolones.
7. Emphasize ciprofloxacin as a commonly used fluoroquinolone.
8. Discuss review and application exercises 12–15 (text, p. 481).

Clinical Laboratory

1. For a group of clients, identify those at risk of developing nephrotoxicity with aminoglycosides.

2. Have students participate in ensuring that blood for peak and trough drug levels is drawn at appropriate times.

3. For all patients receiving a systemic aminoglycoside, have students monitor serum drug levels and renal function tests (e.g., blood urea nitrogen and serum creatinine) for abnormal values.

4. Have students measure fluid intake and urine output and provide other interventions to ensure that a client receiving a systemic aminoglycoside or a fluoroquinolone is well hydrated to preserve renal function and decrease risks of nephrotoxicity.

5. For a client who is receiving a fluoroquinolone, have students assess the reason for use and the client's response (i.e., therapeutic and adverse effects).

TESTBANK QUESTIONS

1. Fluoroquinolones are contraindicated for use with:
   a. gram-negative organisms.
   *b. children.
   c. clients with osteoporosis.
   d. persons over the age of 80.

2. A serious adverse effect of aminoglycosides is:
   a. hypersensitivity reactions.
   b. hepatotoxicity.
   *c. nephrotoxicity.
   d. photosensitivity.

3. An aminoglycoside used preoperatively for bowel sterilization is:
   a. streptomycin.
   *b. neomycin.
   c. tobramycin.
   d. amikacin.

4. Aminoglycosides are primarily used to treat:
   a. hypersensitivity reactions.
   b. tuberculosis.
   *c. gram-negative infections.
   d. AIDS related disorders.

5. Aminoglycosides are used orally to decrease:
   a. serum creatinine levels.
   *b. serum ammonia levels.
   c. gastrointestinal bleeding.
   d. gall stones.

6. The physician orders gentamicin for a child weighing 66 pounds. If the dose range is 6–7.5 mg/kg/day and the child is to receive the medication b.i.d., how many milligrams should the child receive per dose?
   a. 30 mg
   b. 50 mg
   c. 70 mg
   *d. 90 mg

CRITICAL THINKING CASE STUDY

1. Prior to initiating therapy, the client's renal status should be assessed. During treatment, the nurse should be observing for symptoms of nephrotoxicity, which include increased creatinine and BUN and decreased urinary output.

2. An acceptable urinary output is 30 cc/hr, but given the high incidence of renal toxicity associated with aminoglycoside use, you should also assess 24-hour intakes and outputs, vital signs, weight, and lab values. If there is a significant drop in output or another assessment is deviated, you should contact the physician.

3. There is increased risk of nephrotoxicity with concurrent use of aminoglycosides and diuretics. Therefore, you need to check with the physician before you administer the antibiotic. Lasix needs to be administered slowly, and you need to continue to assess the client's renal status.

36
Tetracyclines, Sulfonamides, and Urinary Agents

MAJOR TOPICS

Types of infections for which tetracyclines are used
Contraindications for tetracyclines
Uses of sulfonamides
Drug therapy of urinary tract infections

DRUG LIST

Doxycycline (Vibramycin)
Nitrofurantoin (Macrobid)
Tetracycline (Sumycin)
Trimethoprim/sulfamethoxazole (Bactrim, Septra)

OBJECTIVES

1. Discuss major characteristics and clinical uses of tetracyclines.
2. Recognize doxycycline as the only tetracycline safe for use in clients with renal failure.
3. Discuss characteristics, clinical uses, adverse effects, and nursing implications of selected sulfonamides.
4. Describe nonpharmacologic interventions to prevent and treat urinary tract infections.
5. Recognize trimethoprim/sulfamethoxazole as a combination drug that is commonly used for urinary tract and systemic infections.
6. Describe the use of urinary antiseptics in the treatment of urinary tract infections.
7. Teach clients strategies for preventing, recognizing, and treating urinary tract infections.

TEACHING STRATEGIES

Classroom

1. Tetracyclines are used relatively infrequently in most clinical practice settings, and the instructor may wish to provide a handout summarizing main points rather than spending much class time. Note that most standardized pharmacology tests include one or more items about food and drug interactions that decrease absorption of oral tetracyclines.

2. Discuss the reasons that sulfonamides are infrequently used for systemic infections.

3. Discuss review and application exercises (text, p. 493).

Clinical Laboratory

1. For clients receiving an oral tetracycline, have students assess knowledge about correct self-administration (i.e., not taking with certain foods and other drugs).

2. For a client receiving an intravenous tetracycline, check the venipuncture site at least twice daily for phlebitis.

3. For clients receiving a systemic sulfonamide, have students assess intake and output and renal function tests for abnormal values.

4. For clients with a previous, current, or potential urinary tract infection, have students prepare a teaching plan that includes prophylactic and therapeutic interventions.

TESTBANK QUESTIONS

1. Demeclocycline (Declomycin) is used to inhibit the release of:
   *a. ADH.
   b. TSH.
   c. FSH.
   d. ACTH.

2. Tetracyclines:
   a. delay cell wall synthesis.
   *b. inhibit protein synthesis.
   c. alter membrane permeability.
   d. prevent nucleic acid synthesis.

3. Tetracycline is the drug of choice for:
   a. gonorrhea.
   b. Lyme disease.
   *c. Rocky Mountain spotted fever.
   d. typhoid fever.

4. A benefit of doxycycline versus tetracycline is that it has:
   a. fewer adverse effects.
   *b. a longer half-life.
   c. better absorption.
   d. a broader spectrum of activity.

5. A common adverse reaction associated with the use of minocycline is:
   *a. dizziness.
   b. blurred vision.
   c. constipation.
   d. dry mouth.

6. You know that your teaching regarding doxycycline has been effective if the client states, "I will:
   a. avoid products that acidify my urine."
   b. take the medication on an empty stomach."
   *c. avoid direct sunlight."
   d. discontinue the drug and call the doctor if diarrhea occurs."

7. Before starting tetracycline, you should ascertain if the individual is:
   a. diabetic.
   b. allergic to penicillin.
   *c. pregnant.
   d. taking birth control pills.

8. A client is taking Sumycin 250 mg for a sinus infection and is experiencing significant gastric upset. You should advise the client to:
   a. stop taking the medication.
   *b. try taking the medication with some food.
   c. take the medication with a full glass of milk.
   d. take an antacid prior to each dose.

9. Prior to starting drug therapy for a urinary tract infection, you should:
   *a. obtain a urine specimen for culture and sensitivity tests.
   b. obtain an accurate drug history.
   c. determine if the individual, if a woman, is pregnant.
   d. all of the above.

10. An anti-infective agent used for urinary tract infections that should be taken with food or milk to minimize GI upset and enhance absorption is:
   *a. nitrofurantoin (Furadantin).
   b. nalidixic acid (NegGram).
   c. trimethoprim (Proloprim).
   d. methenamine mandelate (Mandelamine).

11. After a positive urine culture, your client is to start trimethoprim/sulfamethoxazole (Bactrim) orally b.i.d. An important nursing measure would be to:
   a. administer with an antacid.
   *b. force fluids.
   c. restrict fluid intake.
   d. administer with folic acid.

12. Your client, who is to be started on trimethoprim/sulfamethoxazole (Bactrim), is receiving chlorpropamide to control his hyperglycemia. You should monitor him for:
   a. hyperglycemia.
   b. hypokalemia.
   c. hyperkalemia.
   *d. hypoglycemia.

13. The nurse will monitor Mr. C. for side effects of trimethoprim/sulfamethoxazole (Bactrim), which include:
    a. chest pain.
    *b. joint pain.
    c. spastic colitis.
    d. hypotension.

14. You know that your client has understood the teaching you have done regarding sulfonamides if she states, "I will:
    a. chew the tablets completely before swallowing them."
    b. disregard any red coloration to my urine."
    *c. drink 2–3 liters of liquid daily."
    d. lie down if tinnitus occurs."

15. To assess for complications of sulfisoxazole therapy, the following laboratory tests should be performed:
    a. ABGs.
    b. Blood culture
    *c. Serum creatinine
    d. Stool for occult blood

CRITICAL THINKING CASE STUDY

1. Assess her knowledge of tetracycline and be sure that she is not pregnant.

2. Discuss how and when to take the medication. Adverse effects should be discussed, specifically photosensitivity.

3. I would ask her if she has been taking her medication every day on an empty stomach. I would also find out what her expectations were of the medication.

4. A sore throat may be indicative of thrush. After examining her throat and lymph nodes, I would decide whether a throat culture was warranted.

37
Macrolides and Miscellaneous Antibacterials

MAJOR TOPICS

Types of infections for which macrolides are used
Erythromycin as a penicillin substitute
Interference of erythromycin with metabolism of other drugs
Selected miscellaneous antibacterial drugs

DRUG LIST

Azithromycin (Zithromax)
Clarithromycin (Biaxin)
Clindamycin (Cleocin)
Dirithromycin (Dynabac)
Erythromycin (Ery-tab, Erythrocin)
Metronidazole (Flagyl)
Teicoplanin (Targocid)
Vancomycin (Vancocin)

OBJECTIVES

1. Discuss characteristics and specific uses of erythromycin and other macrolides.
2. Compare and contrast macrolides with other commonly used antibacterial drugs.
3. Describe the interference of erythromycin with the metabolism of other drugs.
4. Apply principles of using macrolides in selected client situations.
5. Discuss characteristics, indications for use, and precautions for using chloramphenicol, clindamycin, metronidazole, teicoplanin, and vancomycin.
6. Discuss the roles of metronidazole and oral vancomycin in the treatment of pseudomembranous colitis.

TEACHING STRATEGIES

Classroom

1. Discuss uses and effects of macrolide antibiotics.

2. Compare and contrast erythromycin and the newer macrolides.

3. Discuss review and application exercises 1–5 (text, p. 504).

4. Provide a written handout summarizing the main points about the miscellaneous drugs.

5. Discuss the reasons for restricting use of vancomycin.

6. Discuss review and application exercises 7–10 (text, p. 505).

7. Discuss the Critical Thinking Case Study (SG, p. 137).

Clinical Laboratory

1. In a hospital or long-term care facility, the instructor can scan the medication administration record for clients receiving a macrolide; then, assign students to assess clients for therapeutic and adverse effects.

2. In outpatient settings, have students provide verbal and written instructions for correct self-administration of a newly prescribed macrolide.

3. For a client taking a miscellaneous drug, have a student assess the reason for use (including culture and susceptibility reports) and the client's response (i.e., therapeutic and adverse effects).

4. For a group of clients, have students identify those at risk of developing pseudomembranous colitis and how they plan to assess for this condition.

5. In a hospital setting, ask a pharmacist, infectious disease physician, or an infection control nurse about restrictions on the use of vancomycin.

TESTBANK QUESTIONS

1. Erythromycin is the drug of choice for:
   *a. Legionnaire's disease.
   b. AIDS related syndrome.
   c. typhoid fever.
   d. rheumatic fever.

2. Erythromycin is used with neomycin for:
   a. encephalopathy caused by liver cirrhosis.
   *b. bowel sterilization prior to surgery.
   c. gram-negative urinary tract infections.
   d. severe otitis media.

3. You should discontinue clindamycin (Cleocin) and notify the physician promptly if you observe:
   a. output less than input.
   *b. diarrhea with blood and mucus.
   c. decrease in deep tendon reflexes.
   d. respiratory depression.

4. Clindamycin for acne produces fewer side effects when given:
   a. orally.
   *b. topically.
   c. intramuscularly.
   d. intravenously.

5. Azithromycin and clarithromycin are used for the treatment of:
   *a. respiratory infections.
   b. urinary tract infections.
   c. gastrointestinal infections.
   d. skin infections.

6. To increase absorption, azithromycin should be administered with:
   a. meals.
   b. milk an hour before meals.
   *c. 8 ounces of water.
   d. crackers and no fluid.

7. Macrolides are primarily eliminated via the:
   a. kidneys.
   *b. liver.
   c. intestines.
   d. lungs.

8. Chloramphenicol (Chloromycetin) is administered with erythromycin to treat:
   a. rapidly multiplying bacteria.
   b. chlamydial infections.
   c. gram-positive infections.
   *d. resistant *Staphylococcus aureus* infections.

9. Common adverse effects that occur with the administration of erythromycin are:
   a. photosensitivity and elevated BUN.
   b. blood dyscrasias.
   *c. nausea, vomiting, and diarrhea.
   d. sore mouth and black furry tongue.

10. Your client, who weighs 66 pounds, is being treated with erythromycin ethylsuccinate (EES). If the recommended dose is 30 mg/kg/day, how much will he receive per dose if the medication is ordered q.i.d.?
    a. 125 mg
    b. 150 mg
    c. 175 mg
    *d. 225 mg

11. When administering erythromycin to a client in renal failure, the:
    a. dose should be decreased.
    *b. dose will remain the same.
    c. dose will be increased.
    d. drug should not be administered.

CRITICAL THINKING CASE STUDY

1. The assessment would include breath sounds, chest X-ray, vital signs, and a sputum culture if he has a productive cough.

2. Mr. R. should rest and drink lots of fluids. He may be up walking to try and mobilize his secretions. He may use antipyretics to control his fever. Ideally, erythromycin should be taken on an empty stomach, but because it causes stomach upset it may be taken with food if necessary.

3. Ask her if he has tried the medication with food and if he has been able to keep anything down. Also, ask what her husband's pulse rate and temperature are and if he has urinated and how much. If it is apparent that Mr. R. is dehydrated and unable to keep anything down, he should come to the office.

4. If Mr. R is still vomiting after 2 days, ask the physician to change the medication.

38
Drugs for Tuberculosis and Mycobacterium Avium Complex (MAC) Disease

MAJOR TOPICS

Characteristics of tuberculosis infections
Risk factors for developing multi-drug resistant tuberculosis
Drug therapy of tuberculosis

DRUG LIST

Ethambutol (Myambutol)
Isoniazid (INH)

Pyrazinamide
Pyridoxine (vitamin B_6)
Rifampin (Rifadin)

O B J E C T I V E S

1. Describe unique characteristics of tuberculosis (TB) infection.
2. Discuss the increased incidence of TB, especially multi-drug resistant tuberculosis (MDR-TB).
3. Identify populations at high risk of developing TB.
4. List characteristics, uses, effects, and nursing implications of using isoniazid (INH), rifampin, and pyrazinamide.
5. Describe the rationale for multiple drug therapy in treatment of TB.
6. Discuss common problems associated with drug therapy of drug-susceptible TB and MDR-TB.
7. Discuss the use of aminoglycosides and fluoroquinolones in the treatment of MDR-TB.
8. Describe Mycobacterium avium complex (MAC) disease and the drugs used to prevent or treat it.

TEACHING STRATEGIES

Classroom

1. Discuss patient teaching materials available from the local health department.
2. Ask a nurse in the tuberculosis clinic of the local health department to speak to the class about current recommendations for prevention and treatment of TB.
3. Ask students to list nursing interventions to promote compliance with drug therapy regimens. Write the list on a transparency or marker board. Ask students to evaluate each proposed intervention in terms of expected effectiveness, ease or difficulty with implementation, potential cost in money and time, and likely availability of sufficient state or local funds.
4. Ask students to "brainstorm" about possible ways to implement directly observed therapy for various populations (e.g., rural, mentally ill, homeless).
5. Assign review and application exercises (text, p. 517) to be written and turned in for a grade.
6. Discuss the Critical Thinking Case Study (SG, p. 40).

Clinical Laboratory

1. Review agency policies and procedures regarding interventions to protect patients and health care providers from TB infection.
2. Ask a hospital infection control nurse to speak regarding management of patients with suspected or confirmed TB.
3. For hospitalized clients with suspected or known TB, have students review culture and susceptibility reports if available, write or verbally discuss

prescribed drug therapy, describe medical isolation procedures (e.g., during postclinical conference), and discuss any violations of medical isolation procedures observed.

TESTBANK QUESTIONS

1. Drug resistance to antitubercular drugs can develop when:
   a. multiple drugs are used.
   b. drugs are used for longer than one year.
   c. large doses are used.
   *d. a few doses are taken for a short period of time.

2. A person taking INH should avoid the following because it will increase the risk of hepatotoxicity:
   *a. Alcohol
   b. Sodium
   c. Caffeine
   d. Nicotine

3. For those with close contact to a person with meningitis, the drug of choice for prophylaxis is:
   a. INH (Laniazid).
   b. streptomycin.
   *c. rifampin (Rifadin).
   d. para-amino salicylic acid (PAS).

4. Prior to initiating INH therapy, you should ask your client the following question. "Do you have a history of:
   *a. liver disease?"
   b. reaction to antibiotics?"
   c. diabetes?"
   d. hypertension?"

5. The following antitubercular drug should be taken before meals:
   a. Rifampin (Rifadin)
   b. Para-amino salicylic acid (PAS)
   *c. Ethionamide
   d. INH (Laniazid)

6. Symptoms of a neurotoxic reaction to antitubercular drugs include:
   a. decreased color discrimination.
   b. bradycardia and hypotension.
   c. fever and tachycardia.
   *d. vertigo and hearing loss.

7. Your client, who weighs 220 lbs., is to receive 1500 mg of ethambutol daily. If the recommended dose is 15 mg/kg/day, this dose is:
   a. high.
   b. low.
   *c. appropriate.

8. An expected outcome after the administration of antitubercular medication is:
   a. increased weight.
   b. increased appetite.
   *c. decreased fatigue.
   d. improvement in skin test.

9. The recommended length of treatment for a recent converter who does not have TB is:
   a. 10 days.
   b. 3 months.
   c. 6 months.
   *d. 12 months.

10. You are a public health nurse visiting Mr. J., who has advanced COPD. Which of the following symptoms would lead you to believe that he has also developed TB?
    a. Large amounts of sputum
    b. Dyspnea
    c. Cyanosis
    *d. Night sweats

CRITICAL THINKING CASE STUDY

1. She will need to take the medication for a year. She will have a yearly chest X-ray instead of a PPD test.

2. These may be adverse reactions to the medication. She needs to be seen by her physician who will evaluate her and decide whether or not to discontinue the medication.

39
Antiviral Drugs

MAJOR TOPICS

Viruses and viral infections
Types of antiviral drugs
Limitations of antiviral drug therapy

DRUG LIST

Acyclovir (Zovirax)
Amantadine (Symmetrel)
Ganciclovir (Cytovene)
Indinavir (Crixivan)
Lamivudine (Epivir)
Nevirapine (Viramune)
Ritonavir (Norvir)
Saquinavir (Invirase)
Stavudine (Zerit)
Zidovudine (Retrovir)

OBJECTIVES

1. Describe characteristics of viruses and common viral infections.
2. Discuss difficulties in developing and using antiviral drugs.
3. Identify clients at risk of developing systemic viral infections.
4. Differentiate types of antiviral drugs used for herpes infections, human immunodeficiency virus (HIV) infections, influenza A, and respiratory syncytial virus (RSV) infections.

5. Describe commonly used antiviral drugs in terms of indications for use, adverse effects, and nursing process implications.
6. Discuss the rationale for using combinations of drugs in treating HIV infection.
7. Teach clients techniques to prevent viral infections.

TEACHING STRATEGIES

Classroom

1. Lecture/discussion regarding some ways viral infections and antiviral drug therapy differ from bacterial infections and antibacterial drug therapy. (This approach attempts to relate the unknown to the known, because students are likely to be more familiar with antibacterial drugs than with antiviral drugs.)

2. Emphasize those antiviral drugs that students are most likely to encounter in clinical practice.

3. Discuss types, uses, and effects of selected antiviral drugs.

4. With anti-AIDS drugs, discuss the rationale for combination drug therapy.

5. Have students obtain, read, and summarize a journal article related to HIV infection and its treatment. The instructor may require a computer search for appropriate articles or list names of journals likely to contain such articles.

6. If feasible, ask a client with HIV infection or a health care provider who works with AIDS patients to speak to the class regarding the medical, psychosocial, and economic aspects of living with HIV infection.

7. Discuss interventions to preserve kidney function with nephrotoxic antiviral drugs.

8. Discuss review and application exercises (text, p. 533).

9. Assign the Critical Thinking Case Study (SG, p. 142) to be written and turned in for a grade.

Clinical Laboratory

1. In an outpatient setting, have students provide verbal and written instructions to clients receiving an oral antiviral drug.

2. In a hospital setting, assign students to immunocompromised clients who are receiving an intravenous antiviral drug. Once they have had the time and opportunity to assess clients, question them about the factors contributing to each client's immunocompromised status, the viral infection being treated, the administration and adverse effects of the specific antiviral drug, and their planned interventions.

3. For hospitalized clients with HIV infection, discuss agency infection control procedures.

4. For a client with HIV infection, ask a student to interview the client about behaviors of nurses and other health care providers that the client finds helpful or desirable.

5. For hospitalized clients receiving a nephrotoxic antiviral drug, ask students to monitor BUN, serum creatinine, and intake and output for abnormal values.

6. Ask students to identify clients at high risk of influenza infection and discuss the need for annual influenza vaccine, if indicated.

TESTBANK QUESTIONS

1. A client who is receiving ganciclovir (Cytovene) complains of bleeding. You should suspect the following adverse effect of the medication:
   a. Stomatitis
   b. Leukopenia
   *c. Thrombocytopenia
   d. Liver toxicity

2. A vaccine has been developed to prevent all of the following except:
   a. measles.
   b. mumps.
   c. rubella.
   *d. roseola.

3. A student has a rubella titre drawn for her college physical and it is negative. Before administering the rubella vaccine you should ask her the following question:
   a. "Is there a family history of diabetes?"
   *b. "Are you pregnant?"
   c. "Do you have an Rh negative blood type?"
   d. "Have you ever had an asthma attack?"

4. Acyclovir (Zovirax) is effective in treating:
   a. herpes zoster.
   *b. herpes simplex type 2.
   c. herpes simplex type 1.
   d. cytomegalovirus (CMV).

5. An expected outcome when trifluridine (Viroptic) is administered to a client with epithelial keratitis is:
   *a. decreased pain.
   b. decreased tearing.
   c. decreased blinking.
   d. increased depth perception.

6. Infants being treated for RSV with ribavirin (Virazole) will receive it:
   a. orally.
   b. parenterally.
   c. rectally.
   *d. by inhalation.

7. Amantadine (Symmetrel) is useful for the treatment of:
   *a. influenza A.
   b. CMV retinitis.
   c. keratoconjunctivitis.
   d. HIV infection.

8. When administered concurrently with zidovudine (Ritrovir), the following medications will increase the risk of adverse effects:
   a. Anticholinergics
   *b. Antipyretics
   c. Antacids
   d. Anticonvulsants

9. You are to administer acyclovir (Zovirax) intravenously. The recommended dose is 5 mg/kg q8h. Your client weighs 155 lbs. How much medication will you administer per dose?
   a. 150 mg
   b. 250 mg
   *c. 350 mg
   d. 500 mg

10. The following statement by your client with AIDS leads you to believe that he has understood your teaching regarding zidovudine (Retrovir). "This medication
   a. inactivates the virus and prevents recurrence of the disease."
   b. may result in resistant viral strains when repeated treatments are used."
   *c. slows the progression of the disease but does not cure it."
   d. prevents the occurrence of opportunistic infections."

CRITICAL THINKING CASE STUDY

1. This drug does not prevent transmission of the virus. Granulocytopenia and anemia can develop. The drug may need to be stopped temporarily until your bone marrow recovers.

2. Anxiety, Risk for Injury: Recurrent infections, Social Isolation.

3. The medication is administered parenterally, twice a day for 2 to 3 weeks. A maintenance dose is then given once a day for 5 or 7 days a week. The drug will improve your condition but not cure it.

4. Try to find out from him the location and amount of bleeding. If he is hemorrhaging give him some suggestions to stop the bleeding and tell him to call 911. If you perceive that the situation is not serious allow him time to express his feelings.

40
Antifungal Drugs

MAJOR TOPICS

Types of fungal infections
Characteristics of antifungal drug therapy

DRUG LIST

Amphotericin B (Fungizone, Abelcet)
Fluconazole (Diflucan)

OBJECTIVES

1. Describe distinctive characteristics of fungi and fungal infections.
2. Discuss antibacterial drug therapy and immunosuppression as risk factors for developing fungal infections.
3. Describe commonly used antifungal drugs in terms of indications for use, adverse effects, and nursing process implications.
4. Differentiate between adverse effects associated with systemic and topical antifungal drugs.
5. List interventions to decrease adverse effects of IV amphotericin B.

TEACHING STRATEGIES

Classroom

1. Lecture/discussion regarding some ways fungal infections and antifungal drug therapy differ from bacterial infections and antibacterial drug therapy. (This approach attempts to relate the unknown to the known, because students are likely to be more familiar with antibacterial drugs than with antifungal drugs.)
2. Emphasize those antifungal drugs that students are most likely to encounter in clinical practice.
3. Discuss review and application exercises (text, p. 541).
4. Assign the Critical Thinking Case Study (SG, p. 146) to small groups of students, then discuss as a class.

Clinical Laboratory

1. Have students assess all clients receiving a systemic antibacterial drug for signs and symptoms of candidiasis.
2. In an outpatient setting, have students provide verbal and written instructions to clients receiving an oral or topical antifungal drug.
3. In a hospital setting, assign students to clients who are receiving an intravenous antifungal drug. Once they have had the time and opportunity to assess clients, question them about reasons for using the prescribed drug and their planned interventions related to administering and observing effects of the drug.

TESTBANK QUESTIONS

1. A drug used to treat vaginal candidiasis is:
   a. acrisorcin (Akrinol).
   b. tolnaftate (Tinactin).
   *c. terconazole (Terazol).
   d. Nystatin (Mycostatin).

2. Your client, who weighs 132 lbs., is to receive griseofulvin (Fulvicin) 10 mg/kg daily. If she receives 4 doses daily, how much will she receive per dose?
   a. 75 mg
   b. 100 mg
   c. 125 mg
   *d. 150 mg

3. The following is a highly contagious fungal infection that is spread by sharing hairbrushes and towels:
   *a. Tinea capitis
   b. Tinea pedis
   c. Blastomycosis
   d. Histoplasmosis

4. A client receiving steroids complains of a sore mouth. Which additional symptom would lead you to believe that she has oral candidiasis?
   a. Temperature of 103°F
   *b. White patches in the back of her throat
   c. Purulent exudate from her nose
   d. Hairy tongue

5. The following medication may be administered concurrently with amphotericin B to minimize adverse effects:
   a. Propoxyphene (Darvon)
   *b. Acetaminophen (Tylenol)
   c. Propranolol (Inderal)
   d. Furosemide (Lasix)

6. The following statement by your client leads you to believe that she has understood the teaching you have done regarding amphotericin B (Fungizone). "I know that as a result of taking this medication, I can develop a disorder of my:
   a. pancreas."
   b. liver."
   c. kidneys."
   *d. heart."

7. Nystatin (Mycostatin) is ordered for your client as a "swish." How should she take the medication?
   *a. Rinse the mouth, then swallow the medication.
   b. Gargle, then spit the medication out.
   c. Hold it in the mouth continually, moving it back and forth.
   d. Apply it with a swab to the affected areas.

8. The following medication is effective in treating dermatophytosis:
   a. Acisorcin (Akrinol)
   b. Flucytosine (Ancobon)
   c. Natamycin (Natacyn)
   *d. Griseofulvin (Fulvicin)

9. The following statement indicates that your client understands how clotrimazole (Lotrimin) is to be administered. "I will:
   *a. fill the applicator and insert it into my vagina at bedtime."
   b. apply the medication to my perineal area twice a day."
   c. inject one applicator full daily."
   d. insert the medication into my vagina every 4 hours and apply a sterile pad."

10. Fungal infections can occur as a result of taking:
    a. vinegar douches.
    *b. antibiotics.
    c. oral contraceptives.
    d. oral antidiabetic agents.

CRITICAL THINKING CASE STUDY

1. One of the adverse effects of this drug is photosensitivity. If she is working in the sun, she is at risk to burn. To treat fungal infections of the nails, it is best if artificial nails are not applied to the area; it could jeopardize the healing process.

2. Eat regularly to avoid GI upset, and apply sunscreen. Look out for the adverse effects, and notify a physician if you are experiencing any.

3. Knowledge Deficit, Risk for Injury; Adverse Effects of Drugs, Risk for Noncompliance

4. These are possibly symptoms of an adverse effect of the medication. A complete examination should be performed before a decision is made to stop or change the medication.

41
Antiparasitics

MAJOR TOPICS

Protozoal and helminthic infestations
Scabies and pediculosis
Prevention and treatment of parasitic infestations

DRUG LIST

Chloroquine (Aralen)
Mebendazole (Vermox)
Metronidazole (Flagyl)
Permethrin (Nix, Elimite)

OBJECTIVES

1. Describe environmental and other major factors in prevention and recognition of selected parasitic diseases.
2. Discuss assessment and treatment of pinworm infestations and pediculosis in school-age children.
3. Discuss the drugs used to treat Pneumocystis carinii pneumonia (PCP) in clients with acquired immunodeficiency syndrome (AIDS).

4. Teach preventive interventions to clients planning to travel to a malarious area.

TEACHING STRATEGIES

Classroom

1. Emphasize those parasitic disorders that students are likely to encounter.

2. Discuss environmental factors that promote parasitic diseases.

3. Ask a school nurse or pediatric nurse to speak to the class about the incidence and treatment of pinworm and lice infestations.

4. Discuss review and application exercises (text, p. 554).

5. Discuss the Critical Thinking Case Study (SG, p. 145).

Clinical Laboratory

1. For clients with parasitic infestations, have students teach them about preventing recurrences.

2. Assign students to spend a day with a school nurse or with a nurse at a local health department that provides information and prophylactic drugs to overseas travelers.

3. In home care settings, assess for environmental and personal risk factors for developing parasitic disorders and intervene as indicated.

TESTBANK QUESTIONS

1. When treating Giardia infection with metronidazole (Flagyl), you should assess the client for:
   a. tachycardia and hypotension.
   b. oliguria and weight gain.
   c. upper GI bleeding.
   *d. convulsions and paresthesias.

2. Persons using gamma benzene hexachloride (Kwell) should be instructed to avoid excessive applications because the following can occur:
   a. Fatigue, cough, and dizziness
   *b. Tremors, insomnia, and convulsions
   c. Headache, abdominal cramping, and diarrhea
   d. Anorexia, nausea, and vomiting

3. Vaginal trichomoniasis can be treated topically with:
   a. metronidazole (Flagyl).
   *b. Betadine douche.
   c. pyrimethamine (Daraprim).
   d. halofantrine (Halfan).

4. A drug commonly used to prevent the initial occurrence of malaria is:
   *a. chloroquine (Aralen).
   b. quinine sulfate.
   c. metronidazole (Flagyl).
   d. pyrimethamine (Daraprim).

5. After treatment with gamma benzene hexachloride (Kwell) for pediculosis, the child should be inspected for lice for:
   a. 24 hours.
   b. 72 hours.
   *c. 2 weeks.
   d. 1 month.

6. The following instructions should be given to a person starting gamma benzene hexachloride (Kwell):
   a. Soak in a warm tub, apply lotion to all body surfaces, and leave it on for 48 hours.
   b. After a hot shower, apply the lotion 3 times a day for one week.
   *c. After a warm, morning shower, apply the lotion all over; repeat the procedure before bedtime.
   d. Wear gloves when applying the lotion, and keep it away from your perineal area.

7. A client receiving metronidazole (Flagyl) should avoid:
   a. foods high in vitamin C.
   b. caffeine.
   *c. alcohol.
   d. sodium.

8. Your client is receiving pyrimethamine (Daraprim). To prevent anemia associated with this medication, he should increase the following in his diet:
   a. Iron
   *b. Folic acid
   c. B_{12}
   d. Thiamine

9. For a client being treated with atovaquone (Mepron) for *Pneumocystis carinii* pneumonia, a nursing responsibility is to monitor:
   a. cardiac enzymes.
   b. serum potassium level.
   *c. liver enzymes.
   d. PT and PTT.

CRITICAL THINKING CASE STUDY

1. Bathe, then apply scabacide to all body surfaces except your face, head, and scalp. Wear clean clothing and launder all soiled clothing and bed linens. In 12 to 24 hours, bathe again and dress in clean clothing.

2. You can return to work after you have completed a course of treatment. You may want to wear gloves when providing direct client care until there is no doubt that the scabies is gone.

3. If the scabies is not gone after 2 treatments with Kwell, there are other medications available.

VII
DRUGS AFFECTING THE IMMUNE SYSTEM

42
Physiology of the Immune System

MAJOR TOPICS

Body defense mechanisms
Immunity
Immune cells
Immune disorders

OBJECTIVES

1. Review body defense mechanisms.
2. Differentiate cellular and humoral types of immunity.
3. Describe the antigen-antibody reaction.
4. Discuss similarities and differences between inflammation and the immune response.
5. Discuss roles of various white blood cells in the immune response.
6. Describe the functions of cytokines.

TEACHING STRATEGIES

Classroom

1. Assign students to write definitions of key terms (text, p. 557) before class.

2. Emphasize that this content is vital to understanding immune functions and treatment of immune disorders.

3. Show a transparency of normal hematopoiesis and immune cell development (Figure 42-1, text, p. 560; IM, p. 148).

4. Have students write answers to review and application exercises (text, p. 566).

Clinical Laboratory

1. Assign students to care for clients with an immune disorder.

2. Ask students to list and evaluate clients' white blood cell counts and differential reports for indications of increased susceptibility to infection.

TESTBANK QUESTIONS

1. Passive immunity lasts:
   a. one year.
   b. one week.
   *c. a few weeks or months.
   d. two to three years.

2. IgE is responsible for the release of histamine, which can result in:
   a. urinary retention.
   *b. bronchoconstriction.
   c. hypertension.
   d. tachycardia.

3. Which of the following cells are phagocytes?
   a. Erythrocytes
   b. Lymphoid stem cells
   c. Suppressor T cells
   *d. Monocytes

4. Acquired immunity:
   a. occurs when antibodies are formed by the immune system of another person and transferred to the host.
   b. develops within 6 months after birth.
   *c. occurs when foreign substances stimulate production of antibodies.
   d. develops when antibodies are stimulated to produce WBCs.

5. The following is an autoimmune disorder:
   *a. Systemic lupus erythematosus
   b. Addison's disease
   c. Celiac disease
   d. Cystic fibrosis

6. The WBCs that start phagocytosis are:
   a. monocytes.
   b. macrophages.
   c. eosinophils.
   *d. neutrophils.

7. Lymphokines:
   *a. stimulate bone marrow.
   b. inhibit T cell production.
   c. suppress protein production.
   d. stimulate production of antibodies.

8. Cellular injury initiates:
   a. a drop in pH.
   b. protein catabolism.
   c. antigen-antibody reaction.
   *d. the inflammatory process.

9. Suppressor T cells act by:
   a. secreting a toxic substance that kills antigens.
   b. binding to antigens and damaging their cell membranes.
   *c. stopping the immune response.
   d. inhibiting activity of B cells.

10. Interferons:
    a. promote reproduction of cells.
    b. participate in the inflammatory response.
    c. enhance the differentiation of lymphoid cells into lymphocytes.
    *d. interfere with the ability of viruses to replicate.

11. The level of the following immunoglobin drops at 6 months of age:
    *a. IgG
    b. IgA
    c. IgM
    d. IgD

12. Immunizations:
    a. strengthen antigens.
    *b. stimulate an immune response.
    c. help clients develop a tolerance to certain substances.
    d. suppress the number of T lymphocytes.

13. The stress response:
    a. decreases the activity of neurotransmitters.
    *b. increases secretion of cortisol.
    c. decreases hormone production.
    d. increases urine production.

43
Immunizing Agents

MAJOR TOPICS
Active immunity
Passive immunity

DRUG LIST
Diphtheria-tetanus-pertussis vaccine (DTwP and DTaP)
DTwP and HIB combined (Tetramune)
Haemophilus B vaccine (HibTITER, Pedvax HIB, ProHibit)
Hepatitis B vaccine, recombinant (Recombivax HB, EngerixB)
Pneumococcal vaccine (Pneumovax 23)

OBJECTIVES
1. Discuss common characteristics of immunizations.
2. Discuss the importance of immunizations in promoting health and preventing disease.
3. Identify immunizations recommended for adults.
4. Identify immunizations recommended for children.
5. Discuss ways to promote immunization of children.
6. Teach parents about recommended immunizations and record-keeping.

TEACHING STRATEGIES
Classroom
1. Ask students about their attitudes and experiences in relation to immunizations.
2. Review routine immunization of young children or provide a written handout summarizing current recommendations.
3. Discuss desirability and practicality of standards for pediatric immunizations.
4. Divide the class into small groups and have each group brainstorm about ways to teach parents and caregivers to promote immunizations of children. List ideas on a transparency or marker board as each group states them.
5. Have students write answers to review and application exercises (text, p. 584).
6. Discuss the Critical Thinking Case Study (SG, p. 158).

Clinical Laboratory
1. Have students participate in administering immunizations in a physician's office, outpatient clinic, or long-term care facility.
2. Have students participate in teaching community groups (e.g., schoolchildren, parents, senior citizens) about immunizations.
3. Discuss possible approaches to an adult client with chronic lung disease who refuses to take influenza vaccine.

TESTBANK QUESTIONS
1. A preparation of live cowpox virus provides:
   a. natural immunity.
   b. artificial immunity.
   c. active immunity.
   *d. passive immunity.

2. Vaccines are composed of:
   *a. live, attenuated, or dead microorganisms.
   b. cells from human organs.
   c. full strength toxins released by microorganisms.
   d. sterile suspensions of live virus.

3. A client who had a tetanus vaccination 7 years ago may require another if he:
   a. is exposed to airborne pathogens.
   b. lives in an area where there is an increased incidence of disease.
   *c. receives a puncture wound.
   d. develops a predisposing condition.

4. Immune serums are administered:
   a. by inhalation.
   *b. intramuscularly.
   c. subcutaneously.
   d. orally.

5. The serum administered to an Rh negative mother when she delivers an Rh positive baby is:
   a. ISG.
   b. varicella-zoster immune globulin.
   c. pertussis immune globulin.
   *d. RhoGam.

6. A 22-year-old teacher requests an influenza vaccination. The vaccine is contraindicated for this client if she:
   a. has chronic respiratory problems.
   *b. has an elevated temperature.
   c. has renal impairment.
   d. has diabetes mellitus.

7. It is common for children receiving immunization to experience the following adverse reactions:
   a. Arthralgia and enlarged lymph nodes
   *b. Tenderness at injection site and malaise
   c. Weakness and difficulty walking
   d. Respiratory distress

8. The following vaccine is administered to prevent meningitis:
   *a. Pedvax HIB
   b. Recombivax HB
   c. Attenuvax
   d. IPOL

9. Pneumococcal vaccine is recommended for:
   a. all persons.
   *b. persons with chronic cardiovascular disease.
   c. all women after menopause.
   d. persons who frequently travel outside the country.

10. The following immunization is routinely administered at 15 months of age:
    a. Sabin vaccine
    *b. MMR vaccine
    c. DPT vaccine
    d. Immune serum globulin

CRITICAL THINKING CASE STUDY

1. Ask her what kind of a reaction she had and how she treated the reaction.

2. She will require proof of immunizations or a waiver before she can be admitted to school. She will be exposed to childhood illnesses, and if she is unimmunized and contracts an illness she could be out of school for a significant amount of time.

3. Assess her for a fever and any respiratory problems.

4. It is not uncommon for children to have slight swelling at the injection site for a day or two. Give her some Tylenol because it will help with the discomfort. You can also give her a warm bath or apply a warm compress.

44
Immunostimulants

MAJOR TOPICS

Colony stimulating factors (CSFs)
Interferons
Interleukins

DRUG LIST

Aldesleukin (Proleukin)
Filgrastim (Neupogen)
Interferon-alfa-2a (Roferon-a)
Interferon-beta-1b (Betaseron)
Sargramostim (Leukine, Prokine)

OBJECTIVES

1. Describe the goals and methods of enhancing immune functions.
2. Discuss the use of epoetin in the treatment of anemia.
3. Discuss the use of filgrastim in the treatment of neutropenia induced by anticancer chemotherapy.
4. Describe the use of sargramostim in bone marrow transplantation.
5. Describe the adverse effects and nursing process implications of administering filgrastim and sargramostim.
6. Discuss interferons and aldesleukin in terms of clinical uses, adverse effects, and nursing process implications.

TEACHING STRATEGIES

Classroom

1. Because this content is relatively complex, it is especially important that students prepare for class. Assignments may include reading the chapter in the text, writing descriptions of key terms, looking up the listed drugs, and reviewing immune system physiology (Chapter 42 or a physiology text).

2. Lecture/discussion regarding recent developments in this aspect of immunotherapy.

3. Ask students about their experiences with patients likely to receive these drugs (e.g., those with bone marrow transplants or cancer).

4. Have students write answers to the review and application exercises (text, p. 595).

5. Discuss the Critical Thinking Case Study (SG, p. 60).

Clinical Laboratory

1. Assign students to care for clients with a bone marrow transplant, cancer chemotherapy, or AIDS or other immunodeficiency disorder. Ask students to identify potential benefits of immunostimulant drug therapy.

2. Have students administer the listed drugs when opportunities arise.

3. For clients receiving any one of the listed drugs, have students assess for therapeutic and adverse effects.

TESTBANK QUESTIONS

1. An expected outcome after the administration of filgrastim (Neupogen) for a client with cancer is:
   a. increased RBC.
   *b. decreased number or severity of infections.
   c. increased life expectancy.
   d. slowed tumor growth.

2. For which of the following disorders would aldesleukin (Proleukin) be contraindicated?
   a. Hypertension
   b. Diabetes mellitus
   *c. Pulmonary disease
   d. Renal insufficiency

3. The following drug is effective in stimulating the production of leukocytes:
   a. Bacille Calmette-guérin (BCG)
   b. Epoetin alfa (Epogen)
   *c. Filgrastim (Neupogen)
   d. Interferon-alfa-2a (Roferon A)

4. An expected outcome of the administration of epoetin alfa (Epogen) is a red blood cell count of:
   a. 1.5–3.5 million/mm3.
   *b. 4–5.5 million/mm3.
   c. 5.6–7.2 million/mm3.
   d. 7.3–9 million/mm3.

5. The following statement by your client leads you to believe she has understood the teaching you have done regarding interleukin-2 (aldesleukin). "This drug will:
   a. prevent me from developing renal failure."
   b. stimulate bone marrow regeneration."
   *c. inhibit tumor growth."
   d. prevent me from developing viral infections."

6. The following medication is administered after a bone marrow transplant to treat graft failure:
   a. Interferon-alfa-n3 (Alferon N)
   b. Interferon-gamma-1b (Actimmune)
   *c. Sargramostim (Leukine)
   d. Interferon-alfa-2a (Roferon-A)

7. Serious toxicity of aldesleukin (Proleukin) includes:
   a. heart failure
   b. pancreatic dysfunction
   *c. gastrointestinal bleeding
   d. pulmonary fibrosis

8. Aldesleukin (Interleukin-2) is the drug of choice for treating:
   *a. renal cell carcinoma.
   b. bladder cancer.
   c. hairy cell leukemia.
   d. Kaposi's sarcoma.

9. An adverse effect of zidovudine (Retrovir) is a/an:
   a. increased white blood cell count.
   *b. decreased hematocrit.
   c. increased platelet count.
   d. decreased serum glucose level.

CRITICAL THINKING CASE STUDY

1. Discuss with him what will happen during the hospitalization. Also give him information about the medications he will be taking.

2. The client's vital signs, heart sounds, lung sounds, weight, CBC with differential, and platelet count will be monitored.

3. We do not know at this time whether your graft has been successful or not. We will be monitoring you closely to evaluate the effectiveness of the medication and your response to it.

45
Immunosuppressants

MAJOR TOPICS
Autoimmune disorders
Tissue and organ transplantation

DRUG LIST
Azathioprine (Imuran)
Cyclosporine (Sandimmune)
Muromonab-CD3 (Orthoclone OKT3)
Mycophenolate mofetil (CellCept)
Prednisone
Tacrolimus (FK506) (Prograf)

OBJECTIVES
1. Describe general characteristics and consequences of immunosuppression.
2. Discuss general characteristics and clinical uses of the major immunosuppressant drugs.
3. Identify adverse effects of immunosuppressant drugs.
4. Discuss nursing interventions to decrease adverse effects of immunosuppressant drugs.
5. Teach clients, family members, and caregivers about safe and effective immunosuppressant drug therapy.
6. Assist clients and family members to identify potential sources of infection in the home care environment.

TEACHING STRATEGIES

Classroom

1. Ask students about their previous experiences, if any, with clients undergoing transplants or immunosuppressant drug therapy.

2. Lecture/discussion regarding characteristics, indications for use, adverse effects, and nursing process implications of selected drugs.

3. Show a transparency of Figure 45-1 (text, p. 598; IM, p. 149).

4. Discuss the high risks of infection associated with immunosuppressant drug therapy and nursing interventions to prevent infection.

5. Discuss the review and application exercises (text, p. 610).

6. Discuss the Critical Thinking Case Study (SG, p. 162).

Clinical Laboratory

1. For a client receiving an immunosuppressant drug, have students check laboratory reports to monitor therapeutic and adverse drug effects (e.g., blood urea nitrogen and serum creatinine as indicators of renal function in clients receiving cyclosporine).

2. Assign students to administer immunosuppressant drugs to transplant patients and monitor drug effects.

3. Interview a client who has been receiving an immunosuppressant drug for a while to determine drug effects, usual practices to prevent infection and their success rate, the client's perceptions of helpful and nonhelpful behaviors of health care providers, and suggestions for nursing students in caring for similar clients.

TESTBANK QUESTIONS

1. Symptoms of neurotoxicity produced by cyclosporine (Sandimmune) include:
   *a. confusion, hallucinations, and seizures.
   b. tardive dyskinesia.
   c. lethargy and confusion.
   d. numbness and tingling.

2. Cytotoxic antimetabolites:
   a. increase cellular catabolism.
   *b. block cell reproduction.
   c. suppress bone marrow production.
   d. stimulate the antigen-antibody response.

3. Corticosteroids are used as antirejection drugs because they:
   a. increase production of cytokines.
   b. increase numbers of circulating lymphocytes.
   *c. suppress phagocytosis and initial antigen processing.
   d. enhance the differentiation of monocytes to macrophages.

4. Cyclosporine (Sandimmune) is used:
   *a. to prevent graft versus host disease.
   b. prior to transplant to prepare the recipient.
   c. to decrease the WBC count.
   d. to eliminate T cells.

5. Persons using immunosuppressants should avoid:
   a. caffeine and fat.
   b. foods high in potassium.
   c. foods high in vitamin K.
   *d. alcohol and tobacco.

6. You should be aware that immunosuppression with corticosteroids can cause:
   *a. diabetes mellitus.
   b. Addison's disease.
   c. Crohn's disease.
   d. syndrome of inappropriate antidiuretic secretion (SIADH).

7. Which of the following statements by your client, who is receiving immunosuppressive drugs to prevent rejection of a kidney and pancreas, leads you to believe he needs further teaching?
   a. "Blood levels must be drawn regularly to regulate the dose of the medications."
   b. "Once the threat of rejection is over, I will still need to take these medications."
   c. "I will have to be seen by the doctor regularly to be assessed for adverse effects of the drugs."
   *d. "I will never have to worry about diabetes again."

8. Persons receiving cyclosporine (Sandimmune) should be observed for adverse effects of the drug, which include:
   *a. nephrotoxicity.
   b. bone marrow depression.
   c. heart failure.
   d. respiratory distress.

9. Symptoms of nephrotoxicity related to immunosuppressive therapy include:
   a. decreased WBC.
   *b. increased serum creatinine levels.
   c. hallucinations.
   d. decreased serum albumin levels.

10. When methotrexate is used to treat arthritis, the following lab values should be checked regularly:
    *a. CBC and platelet counts
    b. Sodium and potassium levels
    c. Creatinine and BUN levels
    d. Magnesium and phosphate levels

CRITICAL THINKING CASE STUDY

1. Vital signs will be evaluated. Changes could indicate fluid overload or infection. Intake and output and daily weight will be monitored carefully because organ rejection can be heralded by decreased urinary output and weight gain. Elevations in serum creatinine, BUN, and potassium levels would indicate kidney failure.

2. You will take immunosuppressives the rest of your life, and the doses may need to be adjusted from time to time.

3. The adverse effects of prednisone include: fluid retention, elevated blood glucose levels, electrolyte imbalances, and increased risk of infection. Persons receiving cyclosporine should be observed for symptoms of nephrotoxicity.

4. At this point, we do not know whether you will lose your kidney or not. It is not uncommon to dialyze persons who have had transplants. Right now we will watch you very carefully. Your medication may need to be adjusted, and you may need to be dialyzed several times before your kidney starts functioning.

VIII
DRUGS AFFECTING THE RESPIRATORY SYSTEM

46
Physiology of the Respiratory System

MAJOR TOPICS

Structure and function of respiratory tract
Normal respiration
Common respiratory disorders for which drug therapy is often needed

OBJECTIVES

1. Review roles of the main respiratory tract structures in oxygenation of body tissues.
2. Describe the role of carbon dioxide in respiration.
3. List common signs and symptoms affecting respiratory function.
4. Identify general categories of drugs used to treat respiratory disorders.

TEACHING STRATEGIES

Classroom

1. Lecture/discussion, using objectives as an outline.

2. Suggest that students review content in a physiology text, if desired.

Clinical Laboratory

1. Have students assess each assigned client for actual or potential interferences in respiratory functions (e.g., excessive secretions).

2. For hospitalized clients, have students list laboratory (e.g., arterial blood gases, hemoglobin) and other diagnostic test reports of respiratory function and analyze these in terms of nursing process implications.

TESTBANK QUESTIONS

1. The left lung, in contrast to the right lung, has:
   *a. one less lobe.
   b. one more lobe.
   c. the same number of lobes.
   d. two more lobes.

2. Cilia:
   a. produce mucus.
   b. phagocytize bacteria.
   c. contract smooth muscle.
   *d. move mucus to the larynx.

3. The portion of the respiratory tract that participates in gas exchange is the:
   a. bronchioles.
   b. trachea.
   *c. alveolar sacs.
   d. main stem bronchus.

4. The amount of air inspired and expired with a normal breath (tidal volume) is:
   a. 200–400 cc.
   *b. 500–700 cc.
   c. 800–1000 cc.
   d. 1100–1300 cc.

5. Hypoxemia is a decrease in:
   *a. pO_2.
   b. saturation.
   c. pH.
   d. pCO_2.

6. Atmospheric air contains:
   *a. 21% O_2.
   b. 35% O_2.
   c. 40% O_2.
   d. 50% O_2.

7. A person normally breathes:
   a. 8–14 times per minute.
   *b. 16–20 times per minute.
   c. 22–28 times per minute.
   d. 28–34 times per minute.

8. Ventilation in the lung is affected by:
   a. perfusion.
   b. compliance.
   c. airway patency.
   *d. all of the above.

9. The rate and depth of respiration are controlled by the respiratory center in the:
   a. cerebrum.
   b. cerebellum.
   *c. medulla oblongata.
   d. foramen magnum.

10. In a healthy individual, the respiratory center is stimulated by changes in:
    *a. pCO_2.
    b. pO_2.
    c. pH.
    d. Na+.

11. A deep breath or sigh occurs:
    a. 1–2 times per hour.
    b. 3–5 times per hour.
    *c. 6–10 times per hour.
    d. 12–15 times per hour.

12. Which of the following can increase the respiratory rate?
    *a. Pain
    b. Malnutrition
    c. Elevated blood glucose levels
    d. Gastric over-distention

47
Bronchodilating and Antiasthmatic Drugs

MAJOR TOPICS

Asthma
Chronic obstructive pulmonary disease
Types of bronchodilating medications

DRUG LIST

Albuterol (Proventil, Ventolin)
Beclomethasone (Vanceril)
Cromolyn (Intal)
Epinephrine (Adrenalin)
Ipratropium (Atrovent)
Salmeterol (Serevent)
Theophylline (TheoDur, aminophylline, others)

OBJECTIVES

1. Differentiate the types of bronchodilating drugs and their mechanisms of action.
2. Review effects of adrenergic drugs, including consequences of overuse.
3. List advantages of inhaled beta$_2$-adrenergic agonists over systemic, nonselective adrenergic drugs.
4. Differentiate between short-acting and long-acting inhaled beta$_2$-adrenergic agonists in terms of uses and nursing process implications.
5. Describe theophylline preparations in terms of indications for use, routes of administration, adverse effects, and nursing process implications.
6. Compare adrenergic and xanthine bronchodilators in terms of therapeutic and adverse effects and nursing process implications.
7. Discuss the roles of leukotriene inhibitors, mast cell stabilizers, and corticosteroids in the treatment of bronchial asthma.
8. State the rationale for using inhaled corticosteroids in the long-term treatment of bronchoconstrictive respiratory disorders.
9. Discuss principles of therapy and nursing process for a client with an acute asthma attack.
10. Discuss principles of therapy and nursing process for a client with chronic bronchoconstrictive disease.
11. Describe important elements of using antiasthmatic drugs in children and older adults.

TEACHING STRATEGIES

Classroom

1. Show a transparency of the main pathophysiologic characteristics of asthma (IM, p. 150) and relate these characteristics to the types of drugs used for treatment.

2. Show a transparency of types of antiasthmatic drugs (IM, p. 150).

3. Lecture/discussion, using the objectives as an outline.

4. Ask students about their experiences with clients receiving medications by oral inhalation.

5. Discuss review and application exercises (text, p. 629), or have students complete as a written assignment.

Clinical Laboratory

1. For clients with asthma or other bronchoconstrictive disorders, assign students to assess respiration, administer bronchodilating drugs by oral, inhalation, or intravenous routes, and observe for therapeutic and adverse effects of the drugs.

2. For students assigned to clients with asthma or other bronchoconstrictive disorders, question them about assessment data, nursing diagnoses, goals, and planned interventions and evaluation.

3. Ask students to report serum theophylline levels and to describe how they will use the information in their nursing care.

4. Have students teach clients about antiasthmatic medications.

5. Have students individualize an agency instruction sheet for a particular client.

TESTBANK QUESTIONS

1. Your client may need to have his dosage of theophylline increased if he:
    a. uses insulin.
    *b. smokes cigarettes.
    c. exercises strenuously.
    d. drinks large amounts of caffeine.

2. D. is started on beclomethasone (Vanceril). You know that D. needs additional teaching if he states:
   a. "I will increase my intake of fluids."
   b. "I will shake the aerosol canister well before using it."
   *c. "I cannot administer a second aerosol medication until 30 minutes after taking this medication."
   d. "I will rinse my mouth and the mouthpiece after each use."

3. R. is taking cromolyn (Intal) for asthma. Which of the following statements made by R. leads you to believe she has understood the teaching you have done?
   a. "If I have an acute attack, I will use the inhaler immediately."
   b. "I will cough after using this medication."
   c. "I will use a nasal decongestant along with this medication to enhance its effects."
   *d. "If I do not see a therapeutic response in a month, my physician may discontinue it."

4. An expected outcome after the administration of xanthine bronchodilators is decreased:
   *a. dyspnea.
   b. pCO_2.
   c. tachycardia.
   d. secretions.

5. When administering intravenous theophylline ethylenediamine (aminophylline), the nurse can expect the client to experience:
   *a. tachycardia.
   b. sedation.
   c. hypotension.
   d. dry mouth.

6. The following drug is not appropriate for the acute treatment of asthma:
   a. Aminophylline
   *b. Cromolyn (Intal)
   c. Proventil
   d. Hydrocortisone

7. Corticosteroids are administered to clients in respiratory failure to:
   a. depress the CNS.
   b. reduce the respiratory rate.
   c. produce bronchodilation.
   *d. reduce inflammation and mucus secretions.

8. Symptoms of hypoxia, which may be treated with bronchodilators, include:
   a. copious secretions.
   b. diminished breath sounds.
   *c. anxiety and tachydysrhythmias.
   d. hypotension.

9. If theophylline is administered in conjunction with erythromycin, how will the dose need to be adjusted? It:
   a. will need to be increased.
   *b. will need to be decreased.
   c. will remain the same.
   d. cannot be given with theophylline.

10. Adrenergic bronchodilators should be used with caution in clients who have:
    a. liver disease.
    b. renal disease.
    c. pulmonary disease.
    *d. heart disease.

11. Ipratropium bromide (Atrovent):
    *a. is used to treat chronic bronchitis and emphysema.
    b. is used for mild to moderate asthma.
    c. produces adverse effects, including nasal congestion and throat irritation.
    d. should be used with caution in clients with impaired hepatic function.

12. Cromolyn sodium (Intal):
    *a. can cause paradoxical bronchospasm with overuse.
    b. is used to treat acute asthma attacks.
    c. requires a large fluid intake for it to be effective.
    d. needs to be refrigerated when it is not being used.

13. Administration of the following medication will not improve airway clearance in clients with COPD:
    a. Steroids
    b. Mucolytics
    *c. Antihistamines
    d. Bronchodilators

14. A client is admitted to the ER with an acute asthma attack. He has just used his albuterol inhaler without effect. After being started on an aminophylline drip, he complains of dizziness, numbness, and tingling in his fingers. These are symptoms associated with:
    a. albuterol (Proventil).
    b. tachycardia.
    *c. hyperventilation.
    d. aminophylline.

15. You observe your client using a metered inhaler. To obtain the maximum benefit from the inhaler, he should:
    a. inhale as soon as the inhaler enters his mouth.
    *b. hold his breath for several seconds after releasing the medication.
    c. administer 3 doses of medication within a 1 minute time frame.
    d. exhale as soon as he compresses the inhaler.

16. Bronchodilators work by:
    a. depressing the sympathetic nervous system.
    b. increasing diuresis.
    c. improving respiratory drive.
    *d. relaxing smooth muscle.

17. Theophylline has the shortest half-life in:
    a. neonates.
    *b. children.
    c. middle-aged adults.
    d. elderly adults.

18. Oral caffeine is used to treat apnea in neonates because of its effect on:
    a. bronchial smooth muscle.
    b. lung compliance.
    *c. the respiratory center.
    d. the diaphragm.

19. After being treated for an acute asthma attack with parenteral theophylline, your client is to be discharged on a short-acting form of the medication. You notice she is having difficulty swallowing the medication. The best instruction you can give her is to:
    a. take the medication with milk.
    b. enclose the medication in a piece of bread.
    *c. sprinkle the capsule on semisolid food, such as ice cream or applesauce.
    d. chew the capsule, then swallow it down with a carbonated beverage.

20. A separate line may be inserted for administration of aminophylline:
    a. because aminophylline will lose its effectiveness if diluted with other medications.
    b. because mixing aminophylline with other medications will cause toxicity.
    c. but this is unnecessary because aminophylline readily mixes with other medications.
    *d. because aminophylline is incompatible with several medications.

CRITICAL THINKING CASE STUDY

1. It would be helpful to know how Jenny had been treating her cold. You should ask her if she had taken any OTC medication because some products contain aspirin which could have precipitated the attack. It would also be helpful to know how she had been using her inhaler, and whether she had used the inhaler before exercising, because overuse can cause bronchoconstriction.

2. Aminophylline is a rapid-acting bronchodilator that quickly relieves dyspnea. Solu-Medrol has an anti-inflammatory effect that decreases the swelling in the airways.

3. Tachycardia is a relatively common side effect of the administration of aminophylline. You should tell Jenny that it is an expected side effect but that you will continue to assess her on a regular basis.

4. When administered concurrently with aminophylline, Tagamet increases the effect of aminophylline. The nurse needs to assess the client for toxic side effects of the medication as well as monitor the theophylline levels.

48
Antihistamines

MAJOR TOPICS
Sources and effects of histamine
Types of histamine receptors

DRUG LIST
Cetirizine (Zyrtec)
Diphenhydramine (Benadryl)
Fexofenadine (Allegra)
Loratidine (Claritin)

OBJECTIVES
1. Delineate effects of histamine on selected body tissues.
2. Identify the effects of histamine that are blocked by histamine₁ receptor antagonist drugs.
3. Describe antihistamines in terms of indications for use, adverse effects, and nursing process implications.
4. Discuss advantages and disadvantages of nonsedating antihistamines.

TEACHING STRATEGIES

Classroom

1. Ask students about their personal use of antihistamines (e.g., Which ones do they take? When do they take them? How do the drugs affect them in terms of their activities of daily living?).

2. Show a transparency of the nonsedating antihistamines (IM, p. 151).

3. Discuss the use of antihistamines by children and older adults.

Clinical Laboratory

1. For hospitalized clients receiving diphenhydramine for sleep, have students assess for anticholinergic effects.

2. For hospitalized clients receiving diphenhydramine to prevent an allergic reaction to a blood transfusion or a diagnostic dye, have students assess for excessive sedation.

TESTBANK QUESTIONS

1. Antihistamines are used for all of the following except:
   a. allergic rhinitis.
   b. pruritus.
   *c. viral infections.
   d. motion sickness.

2. Antihistamines should be used with caution in individuals who have:
   a. Parkinson's disease.
   b. hypertension.
   c. diabetes mellitus.
   *d. prostate hypertrophy.

3. The following condition could contraindicate the use of phenothiazine antihistamines:
   a. Colon cancer
   b. Mitral valve prolapse
   *c. Glaucoma
   d. Peptic ulcer disease

4. Information for a client receiving cyproheptadine (Periactin) includes, "You may experience:
   a. headaches."
   *b. an increased appetite."
   c. an increase in your blood pressure."
   d. a drop in blood glucose levels."

5. Adverse effects that you may see when an elderly man receives antihistamines are:
   a. dizziness and headache.
   *b. urinary retention and constipation.
   c. sore mouth and gingivitis.
   d. diarrhea and abdominal cramping.

6. Diphenhydramine hydrochloride (Benadryl) can be administered for:
   a. an acute asthmatic attack.
   b. depression.
   c. hypertension.
   *d. sedation.

7. The following antihistamine is also effective as an antiemetic:
   a. Astemizole (Hismanal)
   b. Clemastine fumarate (Tavist)
   *c. Hydroxyzine hydrochloride (Vistaril)
   d. Trimeprazine tartrate (Temaril)

8. Mrs. J. is being treated with meclizine hydrochloride (Antivert) for Ménière's disease. Which of the following instructions should you give her?
   a. "Check your pulse daily; this drug can produce an irregular pulse."
   b. "Increase the roughage in your diet; constipation can be a problem."
   c. "Use an antacid with this medication; GI upset is common."
   *d. "Do not drive; this drug can produce drowsiness."

9. An antihistamine that does not produce sedation or decreased mental alertness is:
   a. meclizine hydrochloride (Antivert).
   b. chlorpheniramine (Chlor-Trimeton).
   *c. loratidine (Claritin).
   d. diphenhydramine (Benadryl).

10. Azatadine maleate (Optimine), used for chronic urticaria, is appropriate for:
    a. children under the age of 12.
    b. lactating women.
    c. persons with asthma.
    *d. persons over the age of 65.

CRITICAL THINKING CASE STUDY

1. Antivert was ordered to control your dizziness. Adverse effects include: drowsiness, confusion, dry mouth, anorexia.

2. A calm, stress-free environment may help you avoid or lesson the effects of an attack of vertigo.

49
Nasal Decongestants, Antitussives, Mucolytics, and Cold Remedies

MAJOR TOPICS

Signs and symptoms of respiratory disorders
Types of drugs used to relieve common signs and symptoms
Ingredients in multisymptom cold remedies

DRUG LIST

Dextromethorphan (Benylin DM, others)
Guaifenesin (Robitussin)
Phenylephrine (Neo-Synephrine)
Phenylpropanolamine
Pseudoephedrine (Sudafed)

OBJECTIVES

1. Review decongestant effects of adrenergic drugs.
2. Describe general characteristics and effects of antitussive agents.
3. Discuss the rationale for using combination products in treatment of the common cold.
4. Discuss important elements of using antihistamines in children and older adults.
5. Evaluate OTC cough, cold, and allergy remedies for own or clients' use.

TEACHING STRATEGIES

Classroom

1. Relatively little class time is indicated because most students are likely to be familiar with these drugs from personal use.

2. The instructor can ask students to bring containers of multi-ingredient OTC cold remedies or provide copies of drug labels. Divide the class into small groups and have each group analyze one or more products in relation to the active ingredients (e.g., phenylpropanolamine, dextromethorphan, guaifenesin), whether the amount of each active ingredient contained in the recommended dose is therapeutic, and who should not take the product. In addition, ask whether group members would take the product themselves or recommend it for family and friends and have them state rationales for their answers.

Clinical Laboratory

1. When assessing assigned clients, have students ask whether they use OTC cold remedies. If so, obtain the name of the product, the amount and frequency of use, and the client's perception of therapeutic or adverse effects. Then, use a drug reference to analyze the ingredients and the instructions for use to determine whether the particular client can safely continue to use the product.

2. For clients with a disease process or other drug therapy that is likely to interact adversely with an OTC cold remedy, have students teach about products to avoid or use cautiously and to always read the label before using the product.

TESTBANK QUESTIONS

1. The following is a respiratory stimulant:
   *a. Dopamine (Intropin)
   b. Caffeine
   c. Phenytoin (Dilantin)
   d. Epinephrine (Adrenalin)

2. Clients receiving antitussive agents should:
   a. have a productive cough.
   *b. have little or no mucus in their airways.
   c. receive 200 ml of water after cough syrups and lozenges.
   d. minimize their fluid intake until their coughing has subsided.

3. Narcotic antitussive agents:
   *a. have a low addictive potential.
   b. are the drugs of choice for a client with head trauma.
   c. are used in clients with extreme pain that is aggravated by coughing.
   d. are administered by inhalation to adults.

4. When antitussive therapy is begun, the nurse will expect the duration of the effect to be:
   a. 3–5 hours.
   *b. 4–6 hours.
   c. 8–10 hours.
   d. 2–3 hours.

5. The nurse should instruct a client who will be taking nasal decongestants of the following common adverse effect:
   a. Diarrhea
   *b. Dry mouth
   c. Agitation
   d. Numbness in the chest

6. Decongestants are contraindicated in clients with severe:
   *a. hypertension.
   b. hearing loss.
   c. migraine headaches.
   d. arthritis.

7. The following statement by your client indicates successful client teaching regarding antitussive medications:
   a. "Since the cough syrup is not addictive, I can take it as often as I need it."
   b. "It is best to drink fluids after taking cough syrup to prevent an upset stomach."
   *c. "I may feel drowsy when I take this medication."
   d. "A little wine will help relieve the shakiness caused by the drug."

8. When nasal decongestants are taken too frequently, the following can result:
   a. Nausea
   *b. Rebound nasal congestion
   c. Blurred vision
   d. Headache

9. A common ingredient in OTC antitussive medication for children is:
   a. Dilaudid.
   b. Mucomyst.
   c. codeine.
   *d. dextromethorphan.

10. Mucolytics are administered:
    a. orally.
    b. intramuscularly.
    c. intravenously.
    *d. by inhalation.

CRITICAL THINKING CASE STUDY

1. SSKI and Mucomyst are both expectorants. Mr. Z. should increase his fluid intake, turn, cough and deep breathe (TCDB), and ambulate, if possible, to mobilize his secretions. Mucomyst has an unpleasant taste, so he will want to rinse his mouth after using it. Prednisone is used short-term to decrease inflammation. It can cause GI bleeding, so antacids may be administered with it.

2. Breath sounds will be assessed every shift; congestion should improve daily. Vital signs will be assessed; his temperature should go down. Lab values will also be monitored for blood glucose levels, electrolytes, and WBC count.

3. Encourage him to TCDB and ambulate if possible. Offer him fluids at regular intervals.

4. The nausea could be related to the antibiotics. If he is not vomiting and is able to tolerate the nausea, nothing may be done. If the nausea is problematic, an antiemetic can be administered or the antibiotic could be changed.

5. Make sure that you get adequate exercise and rest. Increase your fluid intake and eat a well-balanced diet.

IX
DRUGS AFFECTING THE CARDIOVASCULAR SYSTEM

50
Physiology of the Cardiovascular System

MAJOR TOPICS

Structure and function of the heart, blood vessels, and blood

Overview of cardiovascular disorders usually treated with drugs

OBJECTIVES

1. Review roles of the heart, blood vessels, and blood in supplying oxygen and nutrients to body tissues.
2. Discuss atherosclerosis as the basic disorder causing many cardiovascular disorders for which drug therapy is required.
3. List cardiovascular disorders for which drug therapy is a major treatment modality.
4. Identify general categories of drugs used to treat cardiovascular disorders.

TEACHING STRATEGIES

Classroom

1. Lecture/discussion, using the objectives as an outline.

2. Assign students to study the chapter and write out answers to objectives.

3. Assign students to review content in a physiology text.

Clinical Laboratory

1. Have students assess each assigned client for actual or potential cardiovascular disorders.

2. For hospitalized clients, have students check apical and radial pulses, blood pressure, ECG tracings, laboratory reports, other diagnostic test reports, and prescribed drugs. Then, have them analyze data in relation to possible cardiovascular disorders and nursing process implications.

TESTBANK QUESTIONS

1. The stroke volume is the:
   a. amount of blood returned to the heart.
   b. force with which the heart beats.
   c. degree to which the heart is stretched.
   *d. amount of blood pumped with each heart beat.

2. The structure that lies between the left atrium and left ventricle and permits blood flow during atrial contraction is the:
   a. pulmonary valve.
   *b. mitral valve.
   c. tricuspid valve.
   d. aortic valve.

3. Normal electrical conduction through the heart is:
   a. SA node, bundle branches, AV node, bundle of His, Purkinje's fibers.
   *b. SA node, AV node, bundle of His, bundle branches, Purkinje's fibers.
   c. SA node, bundle branches, AV node, bundle of His, Purkinje's fibers.
   d. SA node, bundle of His, AV node, Purkinje's fibers, bundle branches.

4. The outer layer of the heart is the:
   a. pericardial sac.
   *b. epicardium.
   c. myocardium.
   d. endocardium.

5. The following is true of the heart and the EKG pattern:
   a. The P waves reflect atrial repolarization.
   b. The PR interval represents atrial contraction.
   *c. The QRS complex represents ventricular depolarization.
   d. The T wave represents ventricular depolarization.

6. Cardiac output equals stroke volume times:
   a. preload.
   *b. heart rate.
   c. conductivity.
   d. elasticity.

7. The following blood component helps maintain blood volume by exerting colloid osmotic pressure:
   a. Gamma globulin
   *b. Albumin
   c. Fibrinogen
   d. Leukocytes

8. Erythrocytes:
   a. produce antibodies.
   b. are essential for blood clotting.
   *c. transport oxygen.
   d. function as a defense mechanism against microorganisms.

9. Twenty to thirty percent of all white blood cells are produced by the:
   *a. spleen and lymph nodes.
   b. liver.
   c. bone marrow.
   d. pancreas.

10. The outer layer of the artery is the:
    a. intima.
    b. media.
    *c. adventitia.
    d. atria

51
Cardiotonic–Inotropic Agents Used in Congestive Heart Failure

MAJOR TOPICS

Causes and clinical manifestations of congestive heart failure (CHF)
Effects and toxicity of digitalis

DRUG LIST

Digoxin (Lanoxin)
Digoxin immune fab (Digibind, Digidote)

OBJECTIVES

1. Describe major manifestations of congestive heart failure.
2. List characteristics of digoxin in terms of effects on myocardial contractility and cardiac conduction, indications for use, principles of therapy, and nursing process implications.
3. Differentiate therapeutic effects of digoxin in CHF and atrial fibrillation.
4. Differentiate digitalizing and maintenance doses of digoxin.
5. Identify subtherapeutic, therapeutic, and excessive serum digoxin levels.
6. Identify clients at risk of developing digoxin toxicity.
7. Discuss interventions to prevent or minimize digoxin toxicity.

8. Explain the roles of potassium chloride, lidocaine, atropine, and digoxin immune fab in the treatment of digoxin toxicity.
9. Teach clients ways to increase safety and effectiveness of digoxin.
10. Discuss important elements of using digoxin in children and older adults.

TEACHING STRATEGIES

Classroom

1. Lecture/discussion, using the objectives as an outline.
2. Emphasize digoxin as a commonly prescribed drug that is likely to be encountered in any clinical setting.
3. Have two groups of students debate the desirability of discontinuing digoxin when possible.
4. Have students write answers to the review and application exercises (text, p. 666) outside of class. Provide an opportunity to ask questions or discuss in class.
5. Discuss or have students write answers to the Critical Thinking Case Study (SG, p. 186).

Clinical Laboratory

1. For clients with CHF, have students assess for edema, fatigue, and respiratory distress.
2. For clients receiving digoxin, question students about the reason for use and drug effects.
3. For clients receiving digoxin, have students assess, verbalize, and record the rate and quality of apical and radial pulses.
4. For clients with atrial fibrillation and digoxin therapy, have students analyze 12-lead ECGs or cardiac monitoring strips for drug effects.
5. For clients receiving digoxin, ask students to explain why it is important to monitor for hypokalemia and what they will do if it occurs.

TESTBANK QUESTIONS

1. Digitalis glycosides have a(n):
   a. positive chronotropic effect.
   b. negative dromotropic effect.
   *c. positive inotropic effect.
   d. antihypertensive effect.

2. Identify the expected outcome when milrinone (Primacor) is administered to a client with heart failure:
   a. Improved conduction
   b. Increased heart rate
   c. Decreased blood flow to the coronary arteries
   *d. Greater myocardial contractility

3. The following symptom may indicate that the client is experiencing digoxin toxicity:
   a. Insomnia
   b. Dry mouth
   c. Hypotension
   *d. Visual disturbances

4. Which of the following medications, when administered concurrently with digoxin, will not increase the digoxin level?
   a. Amiodarone (Cordarone)
   *b. Propoxyphene (Darvon)
   c. Quinidine (Quinaglute)
   d. Verapamil (Calan)

5. Amrinone (Inocor) should be used with caution for persons receiving the following medication because hypotension may result:
   *a. Disopyramide (Norpace)
   b. Furosemide (Lasix)
   c. Albuterol (Proventil)
   d. Aspirin

6. Clients with the following disorder should be considered at high risk for developing digoxin toxicity:
   a. Dysrhythmia
   b. Elevated cholesterol level
   c. Diabetes mellitus
   *d. Renal disease

7. Sodium and water retention in heart failure result from the:
   a. action of the sodium-potassium exchange pump in the myocardium.
   b. diminished ventricular filling and compensatory hypotension.
   *c. compensatory action of the kidneys to increase blood volume.
   d. increased cardiac workload.

8. Digoxin does not:
   a. increase the ability of ventricles to empty more completely.
   b. reduce preload.
   c. reduce venous congestion.
   *d. increase end-diastolic pressure.

9. Digoxin's (Lanoxin):
   a. loading dose (digitalization) is 1.2 to 1.6 mg in divided doses over 24 hrs.
   *b. maintenance dose is based on the patient's renal function.
   c. usual route of administration is intramuscular.
   d. onset is 8 to 12 hours.

10. The following factor predisposes a client to digitalis toxicity:
    a. Low serum albumin
    b. Hyperthyroidism
    c. Cardiac function
    *d. Hypokalemia

11. Which of the following statements by your client leads you to believe she has understood the teaching you have done?
    a. "If I miss a dose one day, I will take 2 doses the next day."
    b. "I can take the drug along with my laxative."
    *c. "The drug may be taken with or between meals, but at the same time each day."
    d. "If my pulse is between 50 and 120 beats/minute, then I will take the drug."

CRITICAL THINKING CASE STUDY

1. When a person is being digitalized, a larger than standard dose is administered in 2–3 equal doses. The physician will use M.'s weight to calculate the appropriate dose for M.

2. M.'s pulse rate will drop once she is digitalized. Her heart will beat slower and more efficiently, therefore the symptoms of heart failure should improve. Her urinary output may also increase because of the increased perfusion to her kidneys.

3. The adverse effects of digoxin include dysrhythmias, anorexia, nausea, vomiting, headache, drowsiness, confusion, and visual disturbances. The symptoms of digoxin toxicity are vague and could be misinterpreted as flu symptoms; therefore it is important for M.'s mother to check M.'s pulse and contact the physician if M. has a concurrent pulse change along with other symptoms.

4. Drugs that decrease the effects of digoxin include antacids, cholestyramine, colestipol, laxatives, oral aminoglycosides, barbiturates, and phenytoin. Drugs that increase the effect of digoxin include adrenergic drugs, anticholinergic drugs, calcium preparations, quinidine verapamil, and nifedipine.

5. The physician has ordered daily digoxin levels to determine whether a therapeutic level has been reached. He is also evaluating M.'s electrolytes (K+, Ca+, Mg++) because deviations in those electrolytes can potentiate digoxin toxicity.

6. Blood studies will help establish whether or not medications are being administered. The symptoms of heart failure should improve if the treatment plan is followed.

7. Three nursing diagnoses that would be appropriate for M. include: altered tissue perfusion related to decreased cardiac output, activity intolerance related to decreased cardiac output, and impaired gas exchange related to venous congestion and fluid accumulation.

52
Antiarrhythmic Drugs

MAJOR TOPICS

Normal cardiac conduction
Types of arrhythmias

DRUG LIST

Quinidine
Lidocaine (Xylocaine)

OBJECTIVES

1. Differentiate between supraventricular and ventricular dysrhythmias in terms of etiology and hemodynamic effects.
2. Describe nonpharmacologic measures to prevent or minimize tachyarrhythmias.
3. Discuss the roles of beta-adrenergic blocking agents, calcium channel blockers, digoxin, and quinidine in the treatment of supraventricular tachyarrhythmias.
4. Discuss the effects of lidocaine in the treatment of premature ventricular contractions and ventricular tachycardia.
5. Describe adverse effects and nursing process implications related to the use of selected antiarrhythmic drugs.

TEACHING STRATEGIES

Classroom

1. Lecture/discussion, using the objectives as an outline.
2. Show a transparency of Figure 52-1 (text, p. 669; IM, p. 152) to review the cardiac conduction system.
3. Show a transparency of Figure 52-2 (text, p. 669; IM, p. 153)
4. Show a transparency of the classes of antiarrhythmic drugs (IM, pp. 154–155).
5. Ask a nurse who works in a coronary care unit to speak to the class about arrhythmias that commonly occur after myocardial infarction and how they may be prevented, recognized, or treated.
6. Discuss the Critical Thinking Case Study (SG, p. 192).

Clinical Laboratory

1. Have students compare ECG tracings (from continuous cardiac monitoring or 12-lead ECGs) for a client with an arrhythmia before and after administration of antiarrhythmic drugs.
2. Assign students to care for clients on telemetry units. Ask students to correlate their clinical observations (e.g., vital signs, skin color and temperature, level of consciousness, overall status) with the client's ECG, antiarrhythmic medications, and other objective indicators of cardiovascular functioning.

3. Demonstrate a continuous intravenous lidocaine drip in an emergency or intensive care setting; discuss drug concentration, regulation of flow rate, and how to monitor the client's response.

TESTBANK QUESTIONS

1. Identify how class I drugs affect a client with a dysrhythmia. They:
   a. increase cardiac blood flow.
   b. enhance contractility of cardiac muscle.
   *c. suppress depolarization in cardiac cells.
   d. eliminate ectopic beats.

2. Which adverse effect is associated with the use of calcium channel blockers?
   a. Seeing halos around objects
   b. Hypersalivation
   c. Tachycardia
   *d. Postural hypotension

3. Class I antidysrhythmic drugs are associated with which side effects?
   *a. Prodysrhythmias
   b. Blurred vision and dry mouth
   c. Tinnitus and hearing loss
   d. Pruritus

4. Which of the following drugs will diminish the action of quinidine if given concurrently?
   a. Aspirin
   b. digoxin (Lanoxin)
   *c. Phenobarbital
   d. Tetracycline

5. Which of the following symptoms would suggest that a client receiving lidocaine (Xylocaine) may be experiencing toxicity?
   a. Headache
   b. Nausea
   *c. Confusion
   d. Tachycardia

6. All of class IV antidysrhythmics are:
   a. antihypertensives
   b. nitrates
   c. beta-adrenergic blockers
   *d. calcium channel blockers

7. Bretylium (Bretylol) is used to treat:
   a. heart block.
   b. unresponsive atrial fibrillation.
   c. supraventricular tachycardia.
   *d. ventricular tachycardia.

8. Clients receiving a beta-adrenergic blocker and a calcium channel blocker should be monitored closely for:
   *a. bradycardia.
   b. chest pain.
   c. ventricular dysrhythmias.
   d. bone marrow depression.

9. Sotalol (Betapace) is the only drug that:
   a. causes supraventricular dysrhythmias following a myocardial infarction.
   *b. possesses the characteristics of class II and class III antidysrhythmics.
   c. slows the heart rate and prolongs depolarization.
   d. immediately stops ventricular fibrillation.

10. An adverse effect associated with the use of amiodarone is:
    a. liver failure.
    *b. pulmonary fibrosis.
    c. renal insufficiency.
    d. bone marrow depression.

11. Tachycardia is an adverse effect of:
    a. diltiazem (Cardizem).
    b. bretylium (Bretylol).
    c. tocainide (Tonocard).
    *d. verapamil (Calan).

12. Which of the following information should be given to a client who is receiving amiodarone (Cordarone)?
    *a. Effects take a week or longer.
    b. You may experience lethargy and fatigue.
    c. You will be predisposed to respiratory infections.
    d. You will be predisposed to urinary tract infections.

13. The effect on the ECG that you can expect when a client is receiving verapamil (Calan) is:
    a. sinus tachycardia.
    b. prolonged PR interval.
    c. depressed ST segment.
    *d. widened QRS complex.

14. Drugs that prolong depolarization affect the ECG by:
    a. prolonging the PR interval.
    b. elevating the ST segment.
    c. eliminating U waves.
    *d. increasing the QRS interval.

15. Which of the following drugs is classified as a class IA antidysrhythmic agent?
    a. Acebutolol (Sectral)
    b. Amiodarone (Cordarone)
    *c. Disopyramide phosphate (Norpace)
    d. Bretylium (Bretylol)

16. Quinidine is best tolerated if it is administered:
    a. one hour before meals.
    *b. with meals.
    c. 30 minutes after meals.
    d. at bedtime.

17. The usual dose for a bolus of lidocaine (Xylocaine) is:
    *a. 50–100 mg.
    b. 100–200 mg.
    c. 250–500 mg.
    d. 1000 mg.

18. Which of the following conditions can be exacerbated by the use of moricizine (Ethmozine)?
    a. Hypertension
    b. Anemia
    *c. Arrhythmias
    d. Asthma

19. Clients with diabetes mellitus who are receiving acebutolol (Sectral) must be carefully monitored for:
    a. peripheral neuropathy.
    b. urinary tract infections.
    *c. hypoglycemia.
    d. hyperglycemia.

20. Oral quinidine (Quinaglute) therapy is initiated. The nurse can expect that the client will need to:
    a. see the physician weekly to monitor therapeutic response.
    b. initially have blood levels of quinidine checked daily.
    *c. have regular ECGs.
    d. have continuous ECG monitoring.

21. Your client suddenly develops ventricular tachycardia. The first drug of choice to treat this dysrhythmia is:
    a. esmolol (Brevibloc).
    b. procainamide (Pronestyl).
    *c. lidocaine (Xylocaine).
    d. verapamil (Calan).

CRITICAL THINKING CASE STUDY

1. The usual bolus dose of lidocaine is 1–2 mg/kg, not to exceed 100 mg. If the physician uses Mr. J.'s weight to determine the dosage, he would order between 50 to 100 mg initially, followed by a continuous infusion. The continuous infusion is usually started at 1–2 mg/minute and increased gradually until the PVCs are controlled. Lidocaine is always infused at the lowest possible rate to prevent toxic side effects.

2. If the present dose of lidocaine is not effective, it can be increased to a maximum of 4 mg/minute. Mr. J. should be observed for drowsiness, paresthesias, muscle twitching, convulsions, confusion, urticaria, edema, and anaphylaxis. Adverse reactions are more likely to occur at the higher doses. If Mr. J.'s PVCs are still not controlled, the physician should be notified. The physician has the option of ordering a Pronestyl or bretylium drip to control the PVCs.

3. Mr. J.'s ECG shows first degree heart block. The medication should be dispensed to control cardiac irritability, and the pulse and blood pressure and PR interval should be monitored at regular intervals.

4. After a heart attack, it is normal for people to experience a lack of energy for 4–6 weeks. The ability to climb 2 flights of stairs without becoming short of breath is a good indication that one has enough energy for sexual intercourse. Antiarrhythmic/antihypertensive medications, such as propranolol (Inderal), sometimes have an effect on sexual performance. If you experience a problem, contact your physician.

53
Antianginal Drugs

MAJOR TOPICS

Characteristics and types of angina pectoris
Types of antianginal drugs

DRUG LIST

Diltiazem (Cardizem)
Isosorbide mononitrate (Imdur)
Nifedipine (Procardia, Adalat)
Nitroglycerin (Nitro-Dur, Nitrostat)
Verapamil (Calan)

OBJECTIVES

1. Describe the types, causes, and effects of angina pectoris.
2. Describe general characteristics and types of antianginal drugs.
3. Discuss nitrate antianginals in terms of indications for use, routes of administration, adverse effects, nursing process implications, and drug tolerance.
4. Differentiate between short-acting and long-acting dosage forms of nitrate antianginal drugs.
5. Discuss calcium channel blockers in terms of their effects on body tissues, clinical indications for use, common adverse effects, and nursing process implications.
6. Teach clients ways to prevent, minimize, or treat acute anginal attacks.

TEACHING STRATEGIES

Classroom

1. Lecture/discussion, using the objectives as an outline.

2. Differentiate onset and duration of action with various forms of nitroglycerin (e.g., sublingual tablet, skin patch, intravenous infusion).

3. Ask students if they have cared for clients receiving nitroglycerin. If so, ask how the drug affected the client.

4. Show a transparency of currently approved calcium channel blockers (IM, p. 156).

5. Show a transparency of Figure 53-1 (text, p. 686; IM, p. 157).

6. Show a transparency of cardiovascular indications for use of calcium channel blockers (IM, p. 158).

7. Discuss or assign review and application exercises (text, p. 693).

8. Discuss or assign the Critical Thinking Case Study (SG, p. 196).

Clinical Laboratory

1. For clients on sublingual nitroglycerin, have students ensure that an adequate supply is available within the client's reach.

2. Interview (instructor or a student) a client who takes sublingual nitroglycerin as needed regarding how often the drug is used, how many tablets are taken and how close together, whether relief is obtained, how long it usually takes to obtain relief, whether dizziness or headache occurs, and so forth. This information will help in teaching other clients who are just starting to use sublingual nitroglycerin.

3. For a client who experiences acute angina while being cared for by a student, have the student assess vital signs, activities at onset of chest pain, and interventions that relieve pain.

4. For clients with cardiovascular disease, list the ordered drugs, show the list to students, and ask them to identify any antianginal drugs.

5. Have students locate and read agency instruction sheets regarding nitrates and calcium channel blockers.

6. Have students prepare a teaching plan for a client receiving a nitrate or calcium channel blocker.

TESTBANK QUESTIONS

1. A schedule that would most likely prevent tolerance and maintain a nitrate's effectiveness is:
   a. continuous dosing.
   b. q.i.d. administration.
   *c. an 8 hour nitrate-free period.
   d. a combination of routes.

2. Which of the following medications is not recommended for use in a cardiac arrest situation because it can prolong ischemia?
   a. Epinephrine
   *b. Erythrityl tetranitrate (Cardilate)
   c. Isoproterenol (Isuprel)
   d. Nitroglycerin

3. Decreased pressure in the aorta and carotid sinuses resulting from nitrate therapy may precipitate which of the following complications?
   a. Chest pain
   *b. Tachycardia
   c. Hyperglycemia
   d. Nitrate intolerance

4. Instructions for a client receiving sublingual nitroglycerin should include limiting the number of tablets to 3 at:
   a. 1 minute intervals.
   *b. 5 minute intervals.
   c. 10 minute intervals.
   d. 30 minute intervals.

5. The best advice to give a client who asks how long nitroglycerin may be used once the bottle is opened is:
   a. 1 month.
   b. 3 months.
   *c. 6 months.
   d. 12 months.

6. The following instruction should be given to a client being discharged on nitrates:
   *a. "You will experience headaches, which should subside."
   b. "Discontinue the medication if you become dizzy."
   c. "Take the medication with food or milk."
   d. "Check your pulse before and after taking the medication."

7. All vasodilator drugs decrease oxygen consumption, which should result in decreased:
   a. confusion.
   b. headaches.
   c. heart rate.
   *d. chest pain.

8. Your client is started on an IV drip of nitroglycerin. An adverse effect of the medication that you will be assessing for is:
   *a. hypotension.
   b. arrhythmias.
   c. dyspnea.
   d. cyanosis.

9. Nitrates:
   *a. dilate coronary vessels and redistribute blood flow to ischemic areas in the endocardium.
   b. increase total blood flow in the body.
   c. constrict venous capacitance in systemic circulation.
   d. act by relaxing skeletal muscle, causing vasodilation.

10. To relieve adverse reactions associated with nitroglycerin, you should instruct your client to:
    *a. rest for a brief period after taking nitroglycerin.
    b. take a warm bath.
    c. take an antihistamine.
    d. apply a topical analgesic.

11. Nitroglycerin transdermal patches (Nitro-Dur) are:
    a. a combination of nitroglycerin and digoxin, surrounded by a bandage.
    b. applied once a week to any nonhairy area of the body.
    *c. used when a continuous nitrate effect is desired.
    d. removed before bathing or showering.

12. A common adverse effect of peripheral vasodilators is:
    a. paresthesias.
    *b. flushing.
    c. vomiting.
    d. vertigo.

13. The following statement by your client indicates that she has an adequate understanding of how nitroglycerin is to be administered:
    a. "Once I get a headache, I know a therapeutic drug level has been reached and I will take no more medication."
    *b. "I can take 1 tablet at 5 minute intervals 3 times."
    c. "I can take as much nitroglycerin as I need because it is not habit-forming."
    d. "If I become dizzy, I will stop taking the medication."

14. Beta-adrenergic blockers help to control angina but may cause:
    a. increased blood pressure.
    b. increased force of contraction of the heart.
    *c. decreased oxygen consumption.
    d. reduced activity tolerance.

15. Your client asks you when she can expect relief from chest pain after taking sublingual nitroglycerin. The best answer is:
    *a. 1–2 minutes.
    b. 5–10 minutes.
    c. 15–20 minutes.
    d. 30–60 minutes.

16. Antianginals:
    a. increase the percentage of oxygen absorbed from the blood in the coronary arteries.
    b. increase myocardial oxygen demand.
    *c. increase the supply of oxygen to the myocardium.
    d. decrease the tissues' need for oxygen.

17. Nitroglycerin:
    a. decreases the heart rate.
    *b. dilates the coronary arteries and veins.
    c. increases afterload.
    d. decreases heart muscle contractility.

18. Beta-adrenergic blockers are used for clients with angina because they:
    a. increase the heart rate.
    b. decrease preload.
    c. increase afterload.
    *d. decrease oxygen demand.

19. You should hold your client's propranolol (Inderal) if he develops:
    a. chest pain.
    b. a pulse rate greater than 100.
    *c. systolic blood pressure lower than 90 mm Hg.
    d. diastolic blood pressure higher than 90 mm Hg.

20. Calcium channel blockers:
    a. decrease preload.
    b. increase heart rate.
    c. increase afterload.
    *d. decrease contractility.

21. Calcium channel blockers:
    *a. block the flow of calcium ions into the myocardial cells.
    b. inhibit plasma protein binding.
    c. are excreted unchanged in the feces.
    d. increase smooth muscle contraction.

22. An adverse reaction to a calcium channel blocker is:
    a. agitation.
    *b. heart failure.
    c. confusion.
    d. pulmonary fibrosis.

23. Reflex tachycardia is a common effect when the following drug is administered for angina:
    *a. Nitroglycerin
    b. Propranolol (Inderal)
    c. Atenolol (Tenormin)
    d. Verapamil (Calan)

24. Nitrates alleviate angina symptoms by:
    a. increasing circulating blood volume.
    b. slowing electrical conduction through the heart.
    *c. increasing myocardial oxygen supply.
    d. lowering blood pressure.

25. The nitrate preparation with the longest duration of action is:
    a. sublingual nitroglycerin.
    b. oral nitroglycerin.
    c. nitroglycerin translingual spray.
    *d. nitroglycerin transdermal patch.

CRITICAL THINKING CASE STUDY

1. Mr. D.'s vital signs will be checked every 15 minutes. Tachycardia and hypotension are two common adverse effects of nitroglycerin. Mr. D. must be watched closely because hypotension can decrease blood supply to the coronary arteries, aggravating angina or precipitating a myocardial infarction. Mr. D.'s ECG will be monitored continuously and a complete head to toe assessment will be performed once the chest pain subsides, including an evaluation of his heart sounds.

2. Diltiazem reportedly has the fewest adverse effects of all the calcium channel blockers and is effective in treating angina and will also lower blood pressure. Since Mr. D. experienced undesir-

able side effects from beta-adrenergic blockers, it is better to avoid the beta-adrenergic blocker category of drugs.

3. Headache and dizziness are encountered occasionally along with weakness. Mr. D.'s ECG should be monitored because bradycardia and first degree AV block can occur.

4. Persons taking long-acting nitrates on a regular schedule can develop a tolerance. Many physicians now order long-acting nitrates for 16 hours daily to prevent their clients from developing a tolerance. The adverse effects from nitroglycerin include hypotension, dizziness, and headache. These symptoms can be increased when another antianginal agent is given concurrently. Therefore the two medications should be administered at different times to minimize the adverse effects.

54
Drugs Used in Hypotension and Shock

MAJOR TOPICS

Types of shock
Types of antishock drugs

DRUG LIST

Dobutamine (Dobutrex)
Dopamine (Intropin)
Epinephrine (Adrenalin)
Norepinephrine (Levophed)

OBJECTIVES

1. Identify clients at risk of developing hypovolemia and shock.
2. Identify common causes of hypotension and shock.
3. Discuss assessment of a patient in shock.
4. Describe therapeutic and adverse effects of vasopressor drugs used in the treatment of hypotension and shock.

TEACHING STRATEGIES

Classroom

1. Discuss details of recognition and treatment of anaphylactic or hypovolemic shock. Emphasize that these emergencies may occur in any setting.

2. Have students write answers to review and application exercises (text, p. 701).

3. Assign the Critical Thinking Case Study (SG, p. 198) to small groups for discussion, or have individual students write answers.

Clinical Laboratory

1. For a group of clients, have students identify those with risk factors for developing hypotension and shock.

2. Role-play or conduct a "mock" emergency or rehearsal in which a student finds a client in shock and proceeds with appropriate interventions such as checking vital signs, skin color and temperature, and level of consciousness, calling a physician, bringing emergency drugs and other equipment to the client's location, and so forth.

TESTBANK QUESTIONS

1. The physician has ordered dopamine (Intropin). Which of the following nursing assessments should be a priority?
   a. Monitoring lung sounds
   b. Monitoring bowel sounds
   c. Monitoring heart rate
   *d. Monitoring blood pressure

2. An adverse effect of dopamine (Intropin) that the nurse should be assessing for includes:
   a. hypertension.
   *b. hypotension.
   c. bradycardia.
   d. seizures.

3. Which of the following statements leads you to believe that your client understands why dobutamine (Dobutrex) is being used?
   a. "I am receiving this drug to increase my heart rate and blood pressure."
   b. "This drug will improve my condition."
   *c. "This drug will increase the force of contraction of my heart and increase the blood supply to my major organs."
   d. "They want to slow down my heart rate and decrease my blood pressure."

4. Mr. J. is started on an IV drip of isoproterenol (Isuprel) for hypotension after open heart surgery. An adverse effect you will be assessing for is:
   a. hypertension.
   *b. tachycardia.
   c. bradycardia.
   d. cyanosis.

5. M. has an IV of 200 mg of dopamine (Intropin) in 250 cc of 5% dextrose in water (800 ᴍ g/cc). If the physician wants M. to receive 200 ᴍ g/minute, how fast will you run the IV? (Use microdrip tubing, 1 cc 5 60 gtts.)
   *a. 15 gtts
   b. 30 gtts
   c. 60 gtts
   d. 90 gtts

6. When vasopressor drugs extravasate, the following can result:
   a. Arterial occlusion
   b. Sepsis
   *c. Tissue necrosis
   d. Paresthesia

7. The following statement by your client leads you to believe he has understood the teaching you have done regarding dobutamine (Dobutrex):
   a. "If I continue to have problems once I leave this unit, I can take dobutamine (Dobutrex) orally."
   *b. "They will be monitoring my pulse and blood pressure frequently."
   c. "Severe headaches are common so I will not worry."
   d. "I will not be allowed any oral fluids while I am receiving this medication."

CRITICAL THINKING CASE STUDY

1. Mr. B. weighs 100 kilograms, therefore he should receive between 200–500 ᴍ g/min.

2. You will assess Mr. B. for a decrease in blood pressure, heart rate, urine output, skin temperature, and level of consciousness because all of the aforementioned symptoms are commonly seen in shock and are the result of inadequate perfusion. The severity of the symptoms will determine the course of action.

3. At moderate doses, dopamine increases heart rate, myocardial contractility, and blood pressure. Dobutamine will increase the force of myocardial contraction, and also increase blood pressure when larger doses are given, but it should not induce or contribute to tachycardia, which can increase oxygen demand. The physician is hoping to improve tissue perfusion. If the kidneys are adequately perfused, Mr. B.'s urinary output should increase.

4. Pressor agents may increase oxygen consumption and induce myocardial ischemia. He may also be experiencing pain because hypotension affects perfusion to all major organs. The nurse will continue to monitor Mr. B.'s vital signs and ECG for any changes and will administer O_2 and morphine for the pain along with nitroglycerin. The nurse will encourage Mr. B. to relax. A sedative is usually ordered if a client is extremely anxious.

55
Antihypertensive Drugs

MAJOR TOPICS

Physiology of blood pressure regulation
Characteristics, risk factors, and causes of hypertension
Characteristics and types of antihypertensive drugs

DRUG LIST

ACE Inhibitors

Benazepril (Lotensin)
Captopril (Capoten)
Enalapril (Vasotec)
Fosinopril (Monopril)
Lisinopril (Prinivil, Zestril)
Moexipril (Univasc)
Quinapril (Accupril)
Ramipril (Altace)
Trandolapril (Mavik)

Alpha₁ Blockers

Doxazosin (Cardura)
Terazosin (Hytrin)

Beta Blockers

Atenolol (Tenormin)
Metoprolol (Lopressor)

Calcium Blockers

Amlodipine (Norvasc)
Diltiazem (sustained release) (Cardizem SR, Cardizem CD,
   Dilacor XR)
Nifedipine (sustained release) (Adalat CC, Procardia XL)
Verapamil (Calan, Calan SR, Verelan)

Miscellaneous drugs

Clonidine (Catapres)
Losartan (Cozaar)

OBJECTIVES

1. Describe factors that control blood pressure.
2. Define/describe hypertension.
3. Identify clients at risk of developing hypertension and its sequelae.
4. Discuss nonpharmacologic measures to control hypertension.
5. Review the effects of alpha-adrenergic blockers, beta-adrenergic blockers, and calcium channel blockers in hypertension.
6. Discuss angiotensin converting enzyme (ACE) inhibitors and angiotensin II receptor antagonists in terms of mechanisms of action, indications for use, adverse effects, and nursing process implications.
7. Describe the rationale for using combination drugs in the treatment of hypertension.
8. Describe guidelines for individualizing drug therapy of hypertension.
9. Discuss interventions to increase therapeutic effects and minimize adverse effects of antihypertensive drugs.

TEACHING STRATEGIES

Classroom

1. Lecture/discussion, using the objectives as an outline. The topic of hypertension and its management warrants one or more class periods because of its common occurrence, its potentially serious consequences, the numerous types of drugs used to treat it, and the important role of nurses in drug therapy.

2. Show a transparency of the factors that regulate blood pressure (IM, p. 159).

3. Show a transparency of the major groups of anti-hypertensive drugs (IM, p. 160) and review the mechanism by which each previously discussed group lowers blood pressure.

4. With calcium channel blockers, emphasize that only sustained release forms of diltiazem and nifedipine are approved for treatment of hypertension. In addition, sustained release forms of these drugs are available in different dosage strengths (i.e., diltiazem: 60, 90, 120, 180, 240, and 300 mg capsules; nifedipine: 30, 60, and 90 mg) and with different abbreviations (e.g., Cardizem SR, Cardizem CD, Dilacor XR, Adalat CC, Procardia XL). Emphasize the need for careful comparison of drug orders and available formulations before administration, and emphasize that sustained release forms should not be crushed or chewed.

5. Show a transparency of the mechanism of action of ACE inhibitors (IM, p. 161).

6. Show a transparency of currently approved ACE inhibitors (IM, p. 162). (Note: All but moexipril, a newer drug, were listed in the top 200 outpatient drugs for 1996.)

7. Ask students about their experiences with hypertensive clients or family members.

8. Emphasize the importance of accurate measurement of blood pressure. Ask students if they have observed errors in technique and, if so, to describe the errors.

9. Ask an adult client with hypertension to speak to the class about personal perceptions of the disease, its treatment, and helpful or nonhelpful behaviors of nurses and other health care providers.

10. Noncompliance with drug therapy is a major problem in treating hypertension. Ask students to list possible reasons for noncompliance and possible nursing interventions to promote compliance, as many as they can in 5 or 10 minutes. Then list these on a marker board and discuss as a class (e.g., in terms of the most likely reasons and of ease or difficulty of implementing particular nursing interventions).

11. Ask students to individualize agency or pharmacy instructions for a client on a particular drug.

12. Discuss review and application exercises 9, 10, and 11 (text, p. 719).

13. Assign small groups to discuss the Critical Thinking Case Study (SG, p. 202).

Clinical Laboratory

1. Have students measure blood pressure on all assigned clients and compare the values with previously recorded values.

2. For clients with hypertension, have students assess for personal characteristics and lifestyle habits that may cause or aggravate hypertension and decrease effectiveness of antihypertensive drugs.

3. For clients receiving antihypertensive drugs, have students measure blood pressure before and after administering the drugs. This will help to assess clients' responses to the medications.

4. For clients receiving antihypertensive drugs, identify OTC drugs that can increase or decrease blood pressure.

5. For clients receiving antihypertensive drugs, analyze all prescribed medications for those that may increase or decrease blood pressure.

6. Ask students to identify assigned clients who are receiving a combination of antihypertensive drugs. In postclinical conference, discuss various combinations and clients' responses to the therapy.

TESTBANK QUESTIONS

1. For which of the following problems would a client be ruled out as a candidate for the use of an ACE inhibitor:
   a. Dysrhythmias
   *b. Hyperkalemia
   c. Diabetes mellitus
   d. Hypercalcemia

2. An adverse reaction associated with the use of ACE inhibitors is:
   a. oliguria.
   *b. cough.
   c. elevated hemoglobin levels.
   d. peripheral neuropathies.

3. When ACE inhibitors are added to diuretic therapy as a treatment for hypertension, the result will:
   a. decrease renal blood flow.
   b. produce bradycardia.
   *c. increase vasodilation.
   d. prevent angina.

4. A client using antihypertensive medications needs to know that salt substitutes:
   a. interfere with their action.
   b. may be used liberally.
   c. are unpalatable.
   *d. increase the risk of hyperkalemia.

5. The following medication should be available in case ACE inhibitors produce swelling of the tongue:
   a. Intravenous aminophylline
   b. Intramuscular diphenhydramine
   *c. Subcutaneous epinephrine
   d. Subcutaneous Aquamephyton

6. Peripheral resistance is influenced by:
   a. cardiac output.
   *b. sympathetic nervous system.
   c. smooth muscle tone.
   d. percentage of body fat.

7. The parasympathetic influence on the heart is achieved as a result of:
   a. epinephrine.
   b. norepinephrine.
   *c. acetylcholine.
   d. dopamine.

8. Peripherally acting sympatholytics decrease blood pressure by:
   a. decreasing cardiac output.
   b. enhancing transmission of autacoids.
   c. mediating activity of the baroreceptors.
   *d. inhibiting action of sympathomimetics.

9. The following statement by your client indicates an understanding of an antihypertensive regime:
   a. "If I miss a dose, I will take two at the next dosage time."
   b. "I will take the medication when I feel my blood pressure is high."
   c. "I plan to soak in a hot tub at night to relax."
   *d. "I will not stop taking the drug if I feel dizzy."

10. Your client, who is receiving nitroprusside, develops symptoms such as slurred speech, weakness, muscle twitching, and confusion. You should:
    a. decrease the infusion.
    *b. stop the infusion.
    c. increase the infusion.
    d. start normal saline.

11. An expected outcome of nitroprusside administration is:
    a. reduced cardiac output.
    b. increased preload.
    *c. increased urine output.
    d. increased afterload.

12. Your client is receiving clonidine (Catapres). Prior to initiation of this drug, you will assess for the following condition, which indicates cautious administration:
    a. Migraine headache
    *b. Depression
    c. Glaucoma
    d. Asthma

13. Mr. D. will be taught to be aware of the following side effect related to clonidine therapy:
    a. Restlessness
    b. Anxiety
    c. Diarrhea
    *d. Dry mouth

14. An expected outcome when beta-adrenergic blockers are administered for hypertension is:
    a. increased cardiac output.
    *b. decreased heart rate.
    c. decreased need for diuretics.
    d. increased standing blood pressure.

15. All of the following inhibit the sympathetic nervous system except:
    a. clonidine (Catapres)
    b. methyldopa (Adomet)
    c. atenolol (Tenormin)
    *d. guanethidine sulfate (Ismelin)

16. An antihypertensive drug useful in opiate withdrawal is:
    a. reserpine (Serpasil).
    b. propranolol (Inderal).
    *c. clonidine (Catapres).
    d. Captopril

CRITICAL THINKING CASE STUDY

1. Exercise will help M. lose weight and decrease her blood pressure. A reduction in dietary sodium will also be beneficial for M. Cigarette smoking has been linked to hypertension, so cessation of smoking would be an important goal.

2. Atenolol (Tenormin), a selective beta blocker, is a commonly used first-line antihypertensive medication. Beta blockers will decrease renin levels.

3. M. should have her blood pressure checked at least once a week (some physicians require daily blood pressure checks) while her antihypertensive regime is being evaluated. If her job does not permit her to visit the office on a weekly basis, she could purchase a self-monitoring blood pressure unit and call her blood pressures into her physician. She should be encouraged to keep track of her weight and her dietary intake. A support group such as Weight Watchers may be beneficial.

4. M. was not well-controlled on Inderal. Rather than increase the medication and increase the risk of side effects, the physician changed M.'s medication. In hypertensive clients with renal disease, ACE inhibitors are effective. Diuretics are commonly added to combat the sodium, potassium, and fluid retention that these clients experience.

56
Diuretics

MAJOR TOPICS

Renal physiology
Conditions for which diuretics are used
Types of diuretic drugs

DRUG LIST

Furosemide (Lasix)
Hydrochlorothiazide (HydroDIURIL)
Hydrochlorothiazide/triamterene (Dyazide, Maxzide)
Mannitol (Osmitrol)

OBJECTIVES

1. List characteristics of diuretics in terms of mechanism of action, indications for use, principles of therapy, and nursing process implications.
2. Discuss major adverse effects of thiazide, loop, and potassium-saving diuretics.
3. Identify clients at risk of developing adverse reactions to diuretic administration.
4. Recognize commonly used potassium-losing and potassium-saving diuretics.
5. Discuss the rationale for using combination products containing a potassium-losing and a potassium-saving diuretic.
6. Recognize serum potassium levels that are normal, hypokalemic, or hyperkalemic.
7. Teach clients the importance of taking diuretics and potassium supplements as prescribed.
8. Discuss important elements of diuretic therapy in older adults.

TEACHING STRATEGIES

Classroom

1. Ask students about their experiences with clients receiving diuretics.
2. Remind students that the generic names of all the thiazide diuretics end in "thiazide."
3. For clients receiving diuretics, discuss assessing their conditions for therapeutic and adverse drug effects.
4. Review signs and symptoms of fluid volume deficit.
5. Discuss review and application exercises 6 and 7 (text, p. 732).
6. Discuss the Critical Thinking Case Study (SG, p. 208).
7. Warn students that diuretics are sometimes misused/abused for weight control and discuss the dangers of such use.

Clinical Laboratory

1. For clients receiving a diuretic, have students assess for signs and symptoms of dehydration.
2. For clients receiving a diuretic, have students check laboratory reports for serum potassium level, hematocrit, urine specific gravity, and other indicators of fluid and electrolyte status.
3. Show students a urine sample and ask what conclusions they can draw about the client's hydration status.
4. Have students administer diuretics and observe clients' responses, especially children and older adults.

TESTBANK QUESTIONS

1. After receiving 40 mg of furosemide (Lasix), Mr. J. loses 2.2 lbs (1 kg); this is indicative of a loss of:
   a. 100 ml of body fluid.
   b. 250 ml of body fluid.
   c. 500 ml of body fluid.
   *d. 1000 ml of body fluid.

2. Which of the following instructions would it be important to give to Mr. G. before he is discharged on furosemide (Lasix)? "Take the medication:
   *a. early in the morning."
   b. with milk because it causes an upset stomach."
   c. with a laxative because it causes constipation."
   d. before you go to bed."

3. The following diuretic promotes sodium excretion but saves potassium:
   a. Ethacrynic acid (Edecrin)
   b. Furosemide (Lasix)
   c. Hydrochlorothiazide (HydroDIURIL)
   *d. Spironolactone (Aldactone)

4. Which of the following foods would you encourage clients on loop diuretics to include in their diet?
   a. Ice cream
   *b. Potatoes
   c. Yellow vegetables
   d. Apples

5. Severe fluid overload is commonly treated with:
   a. osmotic diuretics.
   *b. loop diuretics.
   c. potassium-sparing diuretics.
   d. thiazide diuretics.

6. Which of the following medications is classified as a potassium-sparing diuretic?
   *a. Amiloride (Midamor)
   b. Furosemide (Lasix)
   c. Ethacrynic acid (Edecrin)
   d. Chlorothiazide (Diuril)

7. When HydroDIURIL is administered, which of the following laboratory values should be monitored?
   a. Alkaline phosphatase
   b. Blood urea nitrogen levels
   c. Serum chloride levels
   *d. Uric acid levels

8. Clients taking loop diuretics should be observed for:
   a. hyperkalemia.
   b. hyperatremia.
   *c. hypocalcemia.
   d. hypochloremia.

9. Thiazide diuretics are contraindicated in persons with:
   a. emphysema.
   *b. renal failure.
   c. liver failure.
   d. glaucoma.

10. A 12-year-old female with decreased renal function is on furosemide (Lasix). The best indicator of the effectiveness of this medication is:
    *a. her weight.
    b. a statement by the client that she is feeling better.
    c. blood urea nitrogen and creatinine levels.
    d. urinalysis and urine for C and S.

11. Mr. D. is using a diuretic to control his hypertension. Which of the following diuretics would not require him to increase his intake of potassium-rich foods?
    *a. Spironolactone (Aldactone)
    b. Furosemide (Lasix)
    c. Ethacrynic acid (Edecrin)
    d. Hydrochlorothiazide (HydroDIURIL)

12. Drug therapy to decrease cerebral edema for a client with head trauma includes:
    a. prednisone (Deltasone).
    b. furosemide (Lasix).
    *c. mannitol (Osmitrol).
    d. spironolactone (Aldactone).

13. A client is being discharged on a diuretic and potassium supplement. Which of the following statements would indicate the need for further teaching?
    a. "I'll eat a banana if I feel tingling in my hands and feet."
    b. "I'll take my potassium supplement with meals."
    *c. "If I forget my potassium supplement, I will take two tablets the next time."
    d. "I'll steam my vegetables."

14. The physiologic change that a client with heart failure experiences which may necessitate the use of diuretics is:
    *a. decreased blood flow to the kidneys.
    b. constriction of the heart muscle.
    c. increased cardiac output.
    d. decreased pulse rate.

15. A client with mild fluid overload may be treated initially with a(n):
    a. ACE inhibitor.
    b. loop diuretic.
    c. potassium-sparing diuretic.
    *d. thiazide diuretic.

16. Which of the following symptoms would suggest that Mr. P., who is receiving a loop diuretic, is hypokalemic?
    a. Hematuria
    b. Pruritus
    c. Blurred vision
    *d. Muscular pain

17. Which of the following medications may increase potassium loss if administered with a diuretic?
    *a. Prednisone (Deltasone)
    b. Penicillin (Wycillin)
    c. Pentoxifylline (Trental)
    d. Pindolol (Visken)

18. Which of the following electrolyte imbalances is associated with the use of loop diuretics and is manifested by confusion?
    a. Hypocalcemia
    *b. Hyponatremia
    c. Hypokalemia
    d. Hypochloremia

19. Caution should be used when administering thiazide diuretics to clients with:
    *a. diabetes.
    b. hypertension.
    c. osteoporosis.
    d. asthma.

20. When assessing a client with metabolic alkalosis related to administration of loop diuretics, you could find all of the following except:
    a. convulsions.
    b. irritability.
    c. stridor.
    *d. weight gain.

21. A symptom of hypovolemia associated with excessive diuresis includes:
    a. bradycardia.
    *b. hypotension.
    c. anorexia.
    d. tachypnea.

22. Which of the following medications can cause ototoxicity when administered concurrently with a loop diuretic?
    *a. Aminoglycosides
    b. Tetracyclines
    c. Penicillins
    d. Cephalosporins

23. Which of the following statements by your client, who is being treated for heart failure with diuretics, leads you to believe that he has understood your instructions?
    a. "I will limit my carbohydrate intake."
    b. "If I increase my salt intake, I will decrease my fluid intake."
    c. "I will eat small frequent meals."
    *d. "If I gain more than three pounds in one week, I will contact my doctor."

CRITICAL THINKING CASE STUDY

1. Lasix was ordered to diurese Mr. P., resulting in decreased preload, decreased serum potassium levels, and decreased stress on the heart. Aldactone is a potassium-sparing diuretic, which induces fluid loss but retains potassium. Administration of these two drugs cause substantial fluid loss without hypokalemia. Digoxin increases the force of the contraction of the heart and cardiac output.

2. The following assessments should be done: heart rate and rhythm, urinary output, weight, blood pressure, breath sounds, peripheral pulses, and skin temperature.

3. Perform a complete head to toe assessment. If possible, given your facility, get an O_2 saturation. Review all recent lab work and chart data. Have a list of Mr. P.'s medications available, as well as all the assessment information, when you contact his physician.

57
Anticoagulant, Antiplatelet, and Thrombolytic Agents

MAJOR TOPICS
Venous and arterial thrombotic disorders
Blood clotting factors

DRUG LIST
Alteplase recombinant (t-PA) (Activase)
Aspirin
Enoxaparin (Lovenox)
Heparin
Protamine sulfate
Vitamin K
Warfarin (Coumadin)

OBJECTIVES
1. Discuss potential consequences of blood clotting disorders.
2. Compare and contrast heparin and warfarin in terms of indications for use, onset and duration of action, routes of administration, and blood tests used to monitor effects.
3. Discuss nursing process implications of anticoagulant drug therapy.
4. Teach clients on long-term warfarin therapy protective measures to prevent abnormal bleeding.
5. Discuss antiplatelet agents in terms of indications for use and effects on blood coagulation.
6. With aspirin, contrast the dose and frequency of administration for antiplatelet effects with those for analgesic or antipyretic effects and anti-inflammatory effects.
7. Describe thrombolytic agents in terms of indications for use, routes of administration, and major adverse effects.

TEACHING STRATEGIES

Classroom
1. Lecture/discussion, using the objectives as an outline.
2. Show a transparency comparing heparin and warfarin (IM, p. 163).
3. Discuss the nursing care of clients who are receiving heparin and warfarin, including administration, observing responses, and teaching self-administration and monitoring.

4. Identify foods and medications, including OTC products, to be avoided by clients taking warfarin.

5. Review antiplatelet effects of aspirin.

6. Emphasize that most myocardial infarctions are caused by blood clots in the coronary arteries and that thrombolytic agents can limit the extent of infarction if given within a few hours of onset of chest pain.

7. Discuss review and application exercises (text, pp. 746–747).

8. Assign the Critical Thinking Case Study (SG, p. 210) to small groups for in-class discussion or to individual students to write answers.

Clinical Laboratory

1. For clients receiving heparin or warfarin, ask students whether the drug is being given for prophylactic or therapeutic purposes.

2. For clients receiving IV heparin, have students list activated partial thromboplastin time (APTT) results and identify therapeutic values.

3. For clients receiving warfarin, have students list prothrombin time (PT) and international normalized ratio (INR) results, and identify subtherapeutic, therapeutic, or high values and state the nursing process implications of each.

4. For clients who experience excessive bleeding while taking an anticoagulant, ask students what they would assess for (i.e., specific signs and symptoms) and what interventions they would perform.

5. For a hospitalized client being discharged on Coumadin, have a student do the discharge teaching and share the content, format, and teaching techniques with other students during postconference.

TESTBANK QUESTIONS

1. Mr. P. is started on warfarin sodium (Coumadin). When can you expect to see a therapeutic blood level?
   a. 1 hour
   b. 12 hours
   c. 24 hours
   *d. 48–72 hours

2. The physician orders 20,000 units of heparin in 1000 ml of D_5W. The physician wants the heparin to infuse at 500 units per hour. The tubing you have available is 60 gtts per 1 ml. How many gtts will you administer per minute to deliver the correct amount of medication?
   a. 15 gtts/min
   *b. 25 gtts/min
   c. 35 gtts/min
   d. 45 gtts/min

3. A client receiving streptokinase (Streptase) therapy begins to bleed excessively from several sites. Along with stopping streptokinase therapy, the nurse may administer:
   a. protamine.
   b. vitamin K.
   c. intravenous calcium.
   *d. amino caproic acide (Amicar).

4. A client receiving warfarin (Coumadin) for long-term prophylaxis of venous thrombosis should have a prothrombin time (PT):
   a. 1.5–2 times the normal value.
   b. 3–4 times the normal value.
   c. less than normal.
   d. normal; warfarin does not alter PT.

5. Arterial occlusion can be effectively treated with:
   a. dipyridamole (Persantine).
   b. heparin.
   *c. streptokinase.
   d. warfarin (Coumadin).

6. Aspirin inhibits:
   a. the rate of fibrin formation.
   *b. platelet aggregation.
   c. fibrin formation.
   d. the dissolution of clots.

7. An antagonist of warfarin (Coumadin) is:
   a. vitamin A.
   *b. vitamin K.
   c. vitamin B_{12}.
   d. vitamin D.

8. Aminocaproic acid (Amicar):
   a. interferes with fibrin formation.
   b. promotes the dissolution of clots.
   *c. inhibits fibrinolysis.
   d. all of the above.

9. Heparin:
   a. interferes with the formation of a platelet plug.
   *b. inactivates several clotting factors.
   c. interferes with the initial phase of the coagulation cascade.
   d. prevents the synthesis of vitamin K.

10. Warfarin (Coumadin):
   a. is regulated by the partial thromboplastin time (PTT) blood test.
   b. may need to be increased when administered concurrently with enzyme inhibitors.
   *c. will have an increased effect when administered concurrently with sulfonamides.
   d. has a usual maintenance dose of 15 to 20 mg daily.

11. When administering heparin, you should know that:
    a. clotting studies are performed 1 hour before administering each dose of heparin.
    *b. other intramuscular or subcutaneous medications should be avoided.
    c. warfarin (Coumadin) cannot be given concurrently.
    d. the deltoid muscle is the best location for administration.

12. Clients receiving warfarin (Coumadin):
    a. should eat a diet rich in vitamin K.
    *b. will have the drug's dosage regulated by the international normalized ratio (INR).
    c. will be able to use this drug if they are breast feeding.
    d. can continue to use aspirin.

CRITICAL THINKING CASE STUDY

1. You should routinely assess circulation in the extremities (tenderness, redness, swelling, temperature changes, peripheral pulses), as well as pain, vital signs, and breathing.

2. Stay with the client and remain calm. Elevate the head of the bed. Obtain an O_2 saturation if ordered. Administer O_2. If the client is being monitored, get an ECG strip. Contact the physician.

3. M.'s risk factors include sedentary lifestyle, fractured femur, birth control pills, smoking, and possibly peripheral vascular disease secondary to diabetes mellitus.

4. Administer both medications. It takes 2 to 3 days before a therapeutic level of Coumadin is reached.

5. Initially the dose of Coumadin is determined by daily PT levels or INRs. With long-term use, the tests are drawn monthly.

6. M. should avoid foods high in vitamin K and OTC medications containing aspirin. M. should make health care providers aware of the medications that he is using and should carry a medic alert card at all times. Lab tests should be performed on a regular basis.

58
Antilipemics and Peripheral Vasodilators

MAJOR TOPICS

Atherosclerosis
Types of hyperlipoproteinemia
Types of antilipemic drugs

DRUG LIST

Fluvastatin (Lescol)
Gemfibrozil (Lopid)
Lovastatin (Mevacor)
Pentoxifylline (Trental)
Pravastatin (Pravachol)
Simvastatin (Zocor)

OBJECTIVES

1. Discuss the role of hyperlipidemia in the etiology of atherosclerosis.
2. Identify sources and functions of cholesterol.
3. Describe selected cholesterol-lowering drugs in terms of mechanism of action, indications for use, major adverse effects, and nursing process implications.
4. Teach clients nonpharmacologic measures to prevent or reduce hyperlipidemia.

TEACHING STRATEGIES

Classroom

1. Lecture/discussion, using the objectives as an outline.

2. Ask students what they already know about cholesterol.

3. Discuss the review and application exercises (text, p. 757).

Clinical Laboratory

1. Have students list total, LDL, and HDL cholesterol values for several clients. Then, have them analyze the values in terms of risk of cardiovascular disease, whether changes are needed, and how changes can be made.

2. For clients receiving a cholesterol-lowering drug, have students teach ways to increase effectiveness and decrease adverse drug reactions.

TESTBANK QUESTIONS

1. A patient tells you that he is taking cholestyramine (Questran). Because of the undesirable taste, he is mixing the drug with applesauce or fruit juice before swallowing it. This comment indicates to the nurse that the client:
    *a. is taking the drug in an appropriate manner.
    b. needs additional teaching.
    c. may develop diarrhea.
    d. is probably not receiving full benefit from the drug.

2. For a client receiving cholestyramine (Questran), you should instruct him to:
    *a. mix cholestyramine (Questran) with fluids before administration.
    b. double the dose if a dose is forgotten.
    c. eat a diet low in bulk and fiber.
    d. take antilipid agents and other medications at the same time.

3. The following item in a client's history could be a contributing factor to hyperlipidemia:
   a. Poor long-term memory
   *b. High-stress position in a large accounting firm
   c. Rheumatic heart disease as a child
   d. Chronic infections

4. The following represents a contraindication to the use of cholestyramine (Questran):
   *a. Evidence of triglyceride levels about 400 mg/dl
   b. Presence of reduced VLDL levels
   c. History of narrow-angle glaucoma
   d. Use of oral hypoglycemic agents

5. The following statement by your client who is using niacin for hyperlipidemia leads you to believe that he understands the teaching you have done:
   *a. "I will take 1 aspirin 30 minutes before the niacin to minimize flushing."
   b. "If I develop a rash, I will stop taking the drug."
   c. "I will take the medicine on an empty stomach."
   d. "I can only use this medication for 6 months."

6. Following successful therapy with cholestyramine (Questran) you should see a decrease in:
   *a. type IIa hyperlipidemia.
   b. type V hyperlipidemia.
   c. type IV hyperlipidemia.
   d. type III hyperlipidemia.

7. A common adverse effect with cholestyramine (Questran) and colestipol (Colestid) is:
   a. anorexia.
   b. headache.
   *c. constipation.
   d. weakness.

8. Lovastatin (Mevacor):
   *a. decreases hepatic synthesis of cholesterol.
   b. increases the rate of cholesterol catabolism.
   c. decreases hepatic production of triglycerides.
   d. increases oxidation of cholesterol.

9. Pentoxifylline (Trental) improves blood flow by:
   a. decreasing platelets.
   b. increasing vasodilation.
   *c. increasing flexibility of RBCs.
   d. increasing blood viscosity.

10. Clients receiving Trental should be taught to report:
    a. photophobia.
    b. tinnitus.
    *c. bruising.
    d. dysphagia.

11. Discharge instructions for a client receiving Lovastatin (Mevacor) include:
    *a. "Take the medication with food."
    b. "Increase your intake of foods high in vitamin C."
    c. "Avoid food products high in caffeine."
    d. "Drink 12 ounces of water with each dose of the medication."

12. Persons taking pravastatin (Pravachol) should have the following test completed monthly for the first 15 months that they are on the medication:
    a. Pulmonary function
    b. bilirubin levels
    c. serum glucose
    *d. liver function

CRITICAL THINKING CASE STUDY

1. Check for a positive Homan's sign to assess for deep vein thrombosis. Measure the size of each leg so that you can determine whether the edema is increasing or decreasing. Assess for peripheral neuropathy. It is important to document decreased sensation, as well as changes in color, temperature, and skin turgor. Decreased sensation is a safety issue that needs to be addressed. The size, depth, drainage, and specific location of the ulcers needs to be well-documented to help assess improvement or deterioration.

2. Mr. J. has borderline tachycardia, hypotension, and dizziness; all of which are adverse effects of Vasodilan. A blood pressure of 80/60 can affect renal perfusion. Hypotension and dizziness can put a person at risk to fall. Mr. J. should be kept on bedrest until the physician can be contacted.

3. Trental reduces blood viscosity and increases the flexibility of RBCs. Infrequent side effects include dyspepsia, nausea, vomiting, dizziness, and headache. You need to elevate your extremities when you are sitting and attend to your leg ulcers to try and prevent future problems.

X
DRUGS AFFECTING THE DIGESTIVE SYSTEM

59
Physiology of the Digestive System

MAJOR TOPICS

Organs and secretions of the GI tract and accessory organs
Effects of drugs on the GI tract
Effects of GI disorders on drug absorption

OBJECTIVES

1. Review roles of the main digestive tract structures.
2. List common signs and symptoms affecting gastrointestinal functions.
3. Identify general categories of drugs used to treat gastrointestinal disorders.
4. Discuss the effects of nongastrointestinal drugs on gastrointestinal functioning.

TEACHING STRATEGIES

Classroom

1. Assign students to review gastrointestinal physiology independently; provide an opportunity to ask questions.
2. Have students write answers to the review and application exercises (text, p. 764).

Clinical Laboratory

1. For any group of clients, have students list medical diagnoses and prescribed drugs; then, have students identify those diagnoses and drugs associated with adverse effects on the gastrointestinal system.
2. Have students review clients' medical records for results of liver function tests and verbalize or write the nursing implications of any abnormal values.

TESTBANK QUESTIONS

1. The hormone that regulates gastric emptying is:
   a. gastrin.
   b. pepsinogen.
   *c. enterogastrone.
   d. trypsin.

2. The sympathetic nervous system:
   a. decreases gastric secretion.
   *b. slows GI tract function.
   c. increases intestinal motility.
   d. increases intestinal mucus production.

3. The liver:
   a. produces red blood cells.
   b. plays a role in protein catabolism.
   c. synthesizes vitamins A, D, and B_{12}.
   *d. synthesizes cholesterol and clotting factors.

4. The pancreas secretes:
   a. trypsin inhibitor.
   b. sodium bicarbonate.
   *c. glucagon.
   d. chymotrypsin.

5. Gallbladder contraction is stimulated by:
   a. high carbohydrate foods in the stomach.
   b. fat-soluble vitamins in the intestine.
   c. highly acidic foods in the stomach.
   *d. fatty foods in the chyme.

6. Which of the following takes the longest to leave the stomach:
   a. Carbohydrates
   *b. Fats
   c. Proteins
   d. Ethyl alcohol

7. The intrinsic factor is:
   a. necessary for the production of vitamin B_6.
   b. essential for maintaining gastric secretions below a pH of 3.5.
   *c. essential for B_{12} absorption.
   d. produced by Kupffer's cells in the liver.

8. The pancreas produces digestive juice that contains:
   a. trypsin.
   b. chymotrypsin.
   c. amylase.
   *d. all of the above.

60
Drugs Used in Peptic Ulcer Disease

MAJOR TOPICS

Characteristics and causes of peptic ulcer disease
Types of drugs used to treat peptic ulcer disease

DRUG LIST

Aluminum hydroxide/magnesium hydroxide (Mylanta)
Cimetidine (Tagamet)
Famotidine (Pepcid)
Lansoprazole (Prevacid)
Omeprazole (Prilosec)
Ranitidine (Zantac)
Sucralfate (Carafate)

OBJECTIVES

1. Describe the role of Helicobacter pylori and other etiologic factors in peptic ulcer disease.
2. Differentiate the types of antiulcer drugs in terms of their mechanisms of action, indications for use, common adverse effects, and nursing process implications.
3. Describe the similarities and differences of histamine$_2$ receptor blocking agents.
4. Discuss significant drug-drug interactions with cimetidine (Tagamet).
5. Describe characteristics, uses, and effects of selected antacids.
6. Discuss the rationale for using combination antacid products.
7. Teach clients nonpharmacologic measures to manage gastroesophageal reflux disease and peptic ulcer disease.

TEACHING STRATEGIES

Classroom

1. Identify populations at risk of developing peptic ulcer disease.
2. Show a transparency of antiulcer drugs (IM, p. 164).
3. Ask students about their experiences with clients receiving antiulcer drugs.
4. Discuss the pathophysiology of gastroesophageal reflux disease (GERD).
5. Discuss the differences in using histamine$_2$ receptor antagonists for peptic ulcer disease and heartburn.
6. Have students write answers to review and application exercises (text, p. 779).
7. Assign small groups to discuss the Critical Thinking Case Study (SG, p. 223).

Clinical Laboratory

1. For a group of clients, have students identify those at risk for peptic ulcer disease.
2. Have students administer antiulcer drugs and report the procedure and client responses to the clinical group.
3. For a client with a GI drainage tube, have students assess type, amount, and color of any secretions, evaluate them as normal or abnormal, and state nursing interventions needed, if any.

TESTBANK QUESTIONS

1. Antacids treat peptic ulcer disease by:
   a. decreasing gastric secretions.
   b. absorbing gastric hydrochloric acid.
   *c. raising the pH.
   d. combining with the acid to produce alkaline stomach contents.

2. Famotidine (Pepcid) and nizatidine (Axid) are used for the management of peptic ulcers because they:
   *a. decrease the amount and acidity of gastric juices.
   b. inhibit motility and secretions.
   c. stimulate gastric cells to produce pepsin and mucus.
   d. neutralize gastric content.

3. Cimetidine (Tagamet):
   a. is excreted unchanged in the urine.
   b. reduces hydrochloric acid production by 75%.
   c. is administered 3 times a day before meals.
   *d. increases blood levels of theophylline.

4. The following statement by your client taking antacids leads you to believe that she has understood the teaching you have done:
   a. "I will take the medication for life."
   b. "I can use tablets or liquid antacids; the drug effectiveness is the same."
   *c. "If I take antacids with aspirin, it will decrease their effectiveness."
   d. "I will take antacids with meals and at bedtime."

5. Prolonged use of aluminum-containing antacids may cause:
   a. low levels of vitamin B_{12}.
   b. increased production of gastric acid.
   *c. constipation.
   d. hyperphosphatemia.

6. Antacids:
   a. increase the absorption of digitalis products.
   *b. decrease the absorption of tetracycline.
   c. enhance the absorption of propranolol (Inderal).
   d. decrease the effectiveness of ACE inhibitors.

7. The nurse will instruct the client that he may experience the following side effect related to omeprazole (Prilosec) therapy:
   a. Paresthesia
   *b. Abdominal discomfort
   c. Visual disturbances
   d. Cough

8. You are aware that the following is a contraindication to the use of metoclopramide (Reglan):
   *a. Bowel obstruction
   b. Glaucoma
   c. Heart failure
   d. Asthma

9. When administering misoprostol, the nurse will contact the physician if her client experiences:
   a. nausea.
   b. vomiting.
   *c. severe diarrhea.
   d. abdominal discomfort.

10. Your client is started on sucralfate (Carafate). A potential nursing diagnosis would be:
    *a. Alteration in Bowel Elimination: constipation
    b. Risk for Injury: bleeding
    c. Inadequate nutrition due to nausea
    d. Electrolyte imbalance

11. A common side effect related to ranitidine (Zantac) is:
    a. fever.
    *b. headache.
    c. bradycardia.
    d. anxiety.

12. Sucralfate (Carafate) should be:
    a. administered with meals.
    b. crushed and mixed with water.
    *c. given 2 hours before or after other medications.
    d. given along with antacids.

13. A disadvantage related to calcium compounds for neutralizing gastric acid is:
    a. high cost.
    *b. acid-rebound.
    c. secondary hyperphoshatemia.
    d. short duration of action.

CRITICAL THINKING CASE STUDY

1. Mr. J. is given Tagamet because it is a H_2 antagonist. It decreases both the amount and the acidity (hydrogen ion concentration) of gastric juices. It promotes healing, usually within 6–8 weeks. It is also effective in controlling GI bleeding due to peptic ulcer disease.

2. 10 gtts = 1 ml; therefore, in 100 ml there would be 1000 gtts. 1000 gtts ÷ 20 min = 50 gtts/min.

3. The nurse should observe for the following adverse reactions in clients who are using Tagamet: CNS—confusion, dizziness, headache, drowsiness; CV—bradycardia; GI—nausea, diarrhea, constipation, hepatitis; GU—nephritis; DERM—rashes, exfoliative dermatitis, urticaria; ENDO—gynecomastia; HEMAT—agranulocytosis, aplastic anemia, neutropenia, thrombocytopenia, anemia; MS—muscle pain. Drug interactions: there are many.

4. Carafate is a unique drug for short-term treatment of duodenal ulcer. It is a preparation of sulfated sucrose and aluminum hydroxide gel that promotes healing of duodenal ulcers. It combines with ulcer exudate, adheres to the ulcer site, and forms a protective coating that decreases further damage by gastric acid, pepsin, and bile salts. You should assess Mr. J. for constipation and dry mouth.

5. Diet therapy has little role in prevention or treatment of peptic ulcer disease. The client should avoid foods that he finds cause him gastric discomfort. However, the client should be cautioned against using so called "ulcer diets" or bland diets. These diets usually contain large amounts of milk and milk products. Many people consider milk an "antacid" or buffer of gastric acid; however, it has little effect on the pH of gastric juices. Protein and calcium in milk products induce hypersecretion of gastric acid. Thus, a diet regimen that includes milk may actually aggravate peptic ulcer disease. Some suggest that clients should avoid highly spiced foods, gas forming foods, and caffeine containing beverages.

6. Instructions that should be given to Mr. J. before discharge are: Avoid situations that cause or exacerbate symptoms; observe for GI bleeding and other complications of peptic ulcer disease; maintain normal patterns of bowel movements; incorporate relaxation techniques into your lifestyle; continue with course of therapy for 4–8 weeks to ensure ulcer healing; if a dose is missed, take as soon as remembered unless almost time for next dose; do not double doses; cessation of smoking may decrease recurrence of ulcers. Emphasize importance of routine examinations to monitor progress.

61
Laxatives and Cathartics

MAJOR TOPICS

Constipation
Defecation
Types and characteristics of laxatives

DRUG LIST

Bisacodyl (Dulcolax)
Docusate (Colace)
Milk of magnesia
Polyethylene glycol electrolyte solution (CoLyte)
Psyllium (Effersyllium, Metamucil)

OBJECTIVES

1. Differentiate the major types of laxatives according to effects on the gastrointestinal tract.
2. Differentiate the consequences of occasional use from those of chronic use.
3. Discuss rational choices of laxatives for selected client populations or purposes.
4. Discuss bulk-forming laxatives as the most physiologic agents.
5. Discuss possible reasons for and hazards of overuse and abuse of laxatives.

TEACHING STRATEGIES

Classroom

1. This content may be familiar to most students, so that a few minutes may be sufficient to emphasize the main points.
2. Lecture/discussion, using the objectives as an outline.
3. Discuss the review and application exercises (text, p. 787).

Clinical Laboratory

1. For a group of clients, ask students to identify clients with risk factors for developing constipation.
2. Have students assess all assigned clients in relation to bowel elimination. For clients with apparent constipation, have students describe interventions to relieve the condition and to prevent its recurrence.
3. Have students interview clients regarding their use of OTC laxatives (e.g., type, frequency of use) and their willingness to use nondrug interventions.

TESTBANK QUESTIONS

1. Metamucil:
   a. interferes with nutrient and vitamin absorption.
   b. is readily habit forming.
   c. causes bowel evacuation within 20 minutes of ingestion.
   *d. pulls water into the feces, causing expansion
2. Castor oil:
   a. is most effective when administered cold with meals.
   *b. causes a rapid expulsion of contents in the small and large intestine.
   c. is the drug of choice for clients with chronic constipation.
   d. is administered to clients with ulcerative colitis because it coats the bowel lesions.

3. Prior to administering a laxative, you should check for evidence of:
   a. confusion.
   *b. impaction.
   c. heart failure.
   d. urinary incontinence.
4. Persons taking bisacodyl (Dulcolax) should be instructed to expect:
   a. tachycardia and flushing.
   b. low back pain.
   c. blood in their stool.
   *d. severe cramping.
5. Metamucil should be used with caution in clients with:
   a. renal insufficiency.
   b. glaucoma.
   c. hepatic failure.
   *d. diabetes mellitus.
6. You client is receiving magnesium hydroxide (milk of magnesia) PRN every evening; because it has a high sodium and magnesium concentration, you should assess his:
   *a. cardiac status.
   b. liver function studies.
   c. respiratory function.
   d. orientation.
7. Bulk laxatives should be administered with:
   a. oat bran.
   *b. large amounts of fluid.
   c. citrus juice.
   d. unpeeled apples.
8. Clients receiving cascara sagrada should be instructed that it may make their:
   a. urine foul smelling.
   b. breath have a fruity odor.
   c. skin oily.
   *d. urine turn reddish or brown.
9. OTC laxatives such as Ex-Lax contain:
   a. senna.
   *b. phenolphthalein.
   c. mineral oil.
   d. docusate calcium.
10. Magnesium citrate:
    a. takes 4–6 hours before it begins to work
    b. must be followed by a tap water enema prior to a diagnostic test.
    *c. produces a liquid stool and cleanses the bowel.
    d. causes complete bowel elimination with an isotonic saline solution.

CRITICAL THINKING CASE STUDY

1. When Metamucil is administered with small amounts of fluid, it tends to cause constipation rather than act as a laxative.

2. First ask the client if she is uncomfortable. If she has had diarrhea for a number of days and has not eaten a great deal, she may not have a bowel movement for a day or two. Check for bowel sounds and abdominal distention. Give her plenty of hot fluids. If she is uncomfortable, there are glycerin suppositories available at most facilities that do not require a doctor's order. Make sure that she is given an adequate amount of time in the bathroom.

3. A laxative or Dulcolax suppository would be a good place to start. If the aforementioned are not effective, then a Fleet Enema may be necessary. After this problem has been resolved, a stool softener may be helpful.

62
Antidiarrheals

MAJOR TOPICS

Characteristics and causes of diarrhea
Types of antidiarrheal drugs

DRUG LIST

Diphenoxylate/atropine (Lomotil)
Loperamide (Imodium)

OBJECTIVES

1. Identify clients at risk of developing diarrhea.
2. Discuss guidelines for assessing diarrhea.
3. Describe types of diarrhea in which antidiarrheal drug therapy may be indicated.
4. Differentiate the major types of antidiarrheal drugs.
5. Discuss characteristics, effects, and nursing process implications of opiate-related antidiarrheal agents.

TEACHING STRATEGIES

Classroom

1. This content may be familiar to most students, so a few minutes may be sufficient to emphasize the main points.

2. Lecture/discussion, using the objectives as an outline.

3. Discuss the review and application exercises (text, p. 789).

Clinical Laboratory

1. For a group of clients, ask students to identify clients with risk factors for developing diarrhea.

2. Have students assess all assigned clients in relation to bowel elimination. For clients who have diarrhea, have students observe characteristics (e.g., frequency, amount, consistency, and whether mucus, blood, or other abnormal components are present) when possible.

TESTBANK QUESTIONS

1. The following statement by your client leads you to believe your client has understood the teaching regarding pancrelipase. "I will:
   a. take an antacid with this drug one hour before meals."
   *b. not take milk products within an hour of taking this drug."
   c. chew the capsule thoroughly."
   d. take one tablet between meals and at bedtime."

2. When evaluating your client's response to pancrelipase, the following would indicate a need to adjust the medication:
   *a. Steatorrhea
   b. Flatulence
   c. Abdominal cramping
   d. Excessive burping

3. Your client is to receive diphenoxylate hydrochloride (Lomotil) after each diarrhea stool. You should instruct him that he may experience:
   a. anxiety.
   b. bradycardia.
   *c. drowsiness.
   d. urinary retention.

4. A nursing intervention for a client receiving diphenoxylate hydrochloride (Lomotil) is to:
   a. restrict oral fluids.
   b. monitor for bradycardia.
   c. encourage fluids high in potassium.
   *d. assess bowel sounds every shift.

5. Pancreatic enzyme replacement is administered to clients with:
   a. pernicious anemia.
   b. gall bladders that have been removed.
   *c. cystic fibrosis.
   d. insulin-dependent diabetes.

6. A nursing intervention associated with the administration of antidiarrheal adsorbents is:
   *a. Do not administer other medications until 2 hours after the adsorbent.
   b. Administer the adsorbent q.i.d. until there has been no diarrhea for 48 hours.
   c. Discontinue the adsorbent if the stool turns a green color.
   d. Administer adsorbents with large amounts of water.

7. The following statement by your client leads you to believe she has understood your teaching regarding diphenoxylate hydrochloride (Lomotil):
   a. "I am taking this medication because I have infectious diarrhea."
   b. "This drug is used to control colitis."
   c. "Lomotil can be taken indefinitely without worry about tolerance or dependance."
   *d. "It contains atropine and can cause dry mouth and blurred vision."

8. A drug that is effective in treating diarrhea associated with ulcerative colitis is:
   a. tetracycline.
   b. vancomycin (Vancocin).
   c. neomycin.
   *d. sulfasalazine (Azulfidine).

10. An opiate that is effective in treating severe acute diarrhea is:
   a. nalbuphine (Nubain).
   b. propoxyphene (Darvon).
   *c. morphine sulfate.
   d. meperidine (Demerol).

CRITICAL THINKING CASE STUDY

1. Your tumor is causing the diarrhea. We can try to control it with medication, but we cannot eliminate it.

2. You can also eat foods that are constipating: tea, toast, white rice, and bananas.

3. Assess for dehydration, weight loss, and skin breakdown.

4. Morphine will help control his abdominal pain as well as his diarrhea. This is an appropriate dose for a terminally ill client, and it will probably be adjusted upward.

63
Antiemetics

MAJOR TOPICS

Characteristics and causes of nausea and vomiting
Types of antiemetic drugs

DRUG LIST

Cisapride (Propulsid)
Metoclopramide (Reglan)
Ondansetron (Zofran)
Promethazine (Phenergan)

OBJECTIVES

1. Identify clients at risk of developing nausea and vomiting.
2. Discuss guidelines for preventing, minimizing, or treating nausea and vomiting.
3. Differentiate the major types of antiemetic drugs.
4. Discuss the advantages and adverse effects of serotonin receptor antagonists.
5. Discuss characteristics, effects, and nursing process implications of selected antiemetic drugs.

TEACHING STRATEGIES

Classroom

1. Metoclopramide and cisapride can be described together as prokinetic agents, and ondansetron is often used with emetogenic cancer chemotherapy. Most of the other groups of drugs should be familiar to students, so a brief review may be sufficient.

2. Lecture/discussion, using the objectives as an outline.

3. Emphasize the importance of nursing decision-making in administering antiemetic drugs before emetogenic events and PRN.

4. Emphasize that most antiemetic agents cause sedation and that interventions to protect the client may be needed.

5. Discuss the importance of managing nausea and vomiting for clients undergoing emetogenic cancer chemotherapy. This is often a considerable source of anxiety for clients and should be discussed with them prior to starting chemotherapy.

6. Discuss the review and application exercises (text, p. 808).

7. Discuss the Critical Thinking Case Study (SG, p. 231).

Clinical Laboratory

1. For a group of clients, ask students to identify clients with risk factors for developing nausea and vomiting and to provide interventions to prevent occurrence.

2. For clients who have nausea, have students administer prescribed antiemetic drugs and observe clients' responses.

3. For clients who vomit, have students observe and record characteristics (e.g., frequency, amount, and whether undigested food, blood, or other abnormal components are present) when possible.

TESTBANK QUESTIONS

1. Your client is to receive prochlorperazine (Compazine) 30 minutes prior to his scheduled chemotherapy. Before administering the medication you should assess:
   a. pulse.
   *b. blood pressure.
   c. lung sounds.
   d. bowel sounds.

2. Nursing interventions for persons receiving antiemetics for nausea and vomiting should include restricting oral fluids and:
   a. providing small, frequent, high protein meals.
   *b. providing frequent mouth care.
   c. monitoring weights.
   d. encouraging activity.

3. Which of the following statements by Mr. R., who is taking perphenazine (Trilafon), a phenothiazine, indicates the need for further discharge teaching?
   a. "I will get up slowly from a lying position."
   *b. "I can have a glass of wine with my dinner."
   c. "I will refrain from driving a car while I am taking this medication."
   d. "If I have difficulty urinating I will contact my doctor."

4. An extrapyramidal side effect that can occur with large doses of phenothiazines is:
   *a. dyskinesia.
   b. drowsiness.
   c. urinary retention.
   d. hypertension.

5. Which of the following statements by your client, who is receiving dronabinol (Marinol), leads you to believe that he has a good understanding of the effects of this drug?
   a. "This medication is effective for 48 hours."
   b. " It will take several doses before I feel the full therapeutic effects."
   c. "I may experience blurred vision, which will subside 2 hours after administration."
   *d. "This medication has a high potential for abuse."

6. An expected outcome after the administration of antiemetics is:
   a. weight gain.
   b. output greater than intake.
   *c. acid base balance.
   d. hypoactive bowel sounds.

7. The following statement by Mr. G., who will use the Transderm-Scop system for motion sickness, leads you to believe that he has a good understanding of the system:
   a. "I will place the patch on my chest for the best results."
   b. "I will apply the patch when the nausea starts."
   *c. "I know that drowsiness is a side effect of this medication."
   d. "I will remove the patch when I am no longer experiencing nausea."

8. Antiemetics are usually contraindicated in clients with:
   a. glaucoma.
   *b. pregnancy.
   c. duodenal ulcers.
   d. angina.

9. A cannabinoid antiemetic used for persons undergoing chemotherapy and who have not responded to other agents is:
   *a. dronabinol (Marinol).
   b. fluphenazine (Prolixin).
   c. diphenidol (Vontrol).
   d. dimenhydrinate (Dramamine).

10. An example of an OTC antiemetic is:
    a. triflupromazine (Vesprin).
    *b. phosphorlated carbohydrate (Emetrol).
    c. meclizine (Antivert).
    d. metoclopramide (Reglan).

11. When giving cisapride (Propulsid) for nausea, the nurse should observe the client for:
    a. anxiety.
    b. bradycardia.
    c. confusion.
    *d. diarrhea.

12. Besides being used as an antiemetic, meclizine (Antivert) is also effective for the treatment of:
    a. gastric ulcers.
    b. flatulence.
    c. excessive burping.
    *d. vertigo.

13. Antihistamines produce an antiemetic effect by:
    a. blocking dopamine receptors.
    b. stimulating the eighth cranial nerve.
    c. inhibiting local gastric irritations and secretions.
    *d. blocking the action of acetylcholine.

14. An antiemetic drug of choice for children under age 2 is:
    a. scopolamine (Transderm-Scop).
    b. benzquinamide (Emete-Con).
    c. cyclizine (Marezine).
    *d. promethazine (Phenergan).

15. For a client with diabetic gastroparesis, which of the following medications would increase the rate of gastric emptying?
    a. Diphenidol (Vontrol)
    b. Trimethobenzamide (Tigan)
    *c. Metoclopramide (Reglan)
    d. Ondansetron (Zofran)

CRITICAL THINKING CASE STUDY

1. Ativan does not stop nausea, but it decreases the client's memory of nausea. Thus, it helps eliminate anticipatory nausea before a treatment.

2. Small, frequent, high carbohydrate meals may be helpful. Administering antiemetics before a chemotherapy treatment is also helpful.

3. Compazine is a phenothiazine that can be administered intramuscularly or rectally. This drug, a CNS depressant, is considered safe for treating nausea and vomiting associated with chemotherapy, but it can cause drowsiness.

XI
DRUGS USED IN SPECIAL CONDITIONS

64
Antineoplastic Drugs

MAJOR TOPICS
Characteristics of normal and malignant cells
Causes and types of cancer
Types of anticancer drugs

DRUG LIST
Busulfan (Myleran)
Chlorambucil (Leukeran)
Cisplatin (Platinol)
Doxorubicin (Adriamycin)
Etoposide (VePesid)
Fluorouracil (Adrucil)
Methotrexate (Amethopterin)
Tamoxifen (Nolvadex)
Vincristine (Oncovin)

OBJECTIVES
1. Contrast normal and malignant cells.
2. Describe major types of antineoplastic drugs in terms of mechanism of action, indications for use, administration, and nursing process implications.
3. Discuss common and serious adverse drug effects.
4. Describe pharmacologic interventions to prevent or minimize adverse drug effects.
5. Describe nonpharmacologic interventions to prevent or minimize adverse drug effects.
6. Teach clients about their chemotherapy regimens.

TEACHING STRATEGIES

Classroom

1. Emphasize that antineoplastic chemotherapy is best performed by physicians and nurses who specialize in oncology.

2. Show a transparency of major groups of anti-cancer drugs (IM, p. 165).

3. Emphasize individual drugs or groups of drugs that students are likely to encounter in clinical practice.

4. Ask an oncology nurse to speak to the class about the knowledge and skills required in administering anticancer drugs.

5. Have students write answers to the review and application exercises (text, p. 833).

6. Assign the Critical Thinking Case Study (SG, p. 257) to small groups for discussion.

Clinical Laboratory

1. For clients receiving anticancer chemotherapy, have students list drugs, look up unfamiliar drugs in a reference book, and analyze the information to determine potential adverse drug effects. Then, observe and interview clients and review laboratory reports for values indicating adverse drug effects.

2. For clients newly ordered on outpatient intra-venous anticancer drug therapy, teach what to expect in terms of where, when, and by whom medications will be given. Also, teach about possible adverse drug effects and how they can be prevented or managed.

3. For outpatients receiving oral anticancer drugs, have students interview clients regarding attitude toward the medication regimen, any problems associated with the drug therapy, the degree of compliance with the prescribed therapy, and whether health care providers are seen as supportive.

4. Assign students to a day with a nurse in a clinic or physician's office who administers antineo-plastic chemotherapy. Have students write a short description of their observations and feelings about the experience.

TESTBANK QUESTIONS

1. During the S phase of cell division:
   a. the cell rests.
   *b. DNA synthesis occurs.
   c. specialized protein synthesis occurs.
   d. cell mitosis occurs.

2. Cytotoxic drugs are most effective:
   a. against resting cells.
   b. when the tumor is large.
   c. when there is greater organ involvement.
   *d. against dividing cells.

3. Cell cycle nonspecific agents:
   a. are effective against small tumors when growth is rapid.
   b. are given continuously for long periods.
   c. cause a biochemical blockade at the S1 phase of the cell cycle.
   *d. are dose dependent and administered inter-mittently.

4. The dose of antineoplastic agents administered to adults depends primarily on the client's:
   a. weight.
   *b. bone marrow function.
   c. sex.
   d. cardiac function.

5. Prior to administering fluorouracil (Adrucil), you will check the client's:
   a. serum potassium levels.
   b. creatinine clearance.
   *c. white blood cell count.
   d. liver enzymes.

6. An appropriate nursing intervention for a client receiving doxorubicin (Adriamycin) is to:
   a. restrict fluid intake to 2000 ml daily.
   *b. provide frequent oral care.
   c. limit sodium intake to 2000 mg/day.
   d. monitor thyroid studies.

7. Your client is being discharged on cyclophos-phamide (Cytoxan). You know that your teaching has been successful if the client states, "I will:
   a. take Cytoxan with meals."
   b. double the dose if I miss one."
   c. take Cytoxan at bedtime."
   *d. drink plenty of fluids."

8. For a client who has been experiencing nausea, vomiting, and diarrhea after radiation therapy, the most appropriate nursing intervention is to:
   a. administer Imodium and a cup of hot tea immediately after the treatment.
   b. offer crackers before and after the radiation treatment.
   c. encourage the intake of carbonated beverages before the radiation treatment.
   *d. administer an antiemetic 1 hour before the treatment.

9. A priority goal for clients receiving chemothera-py is to:
   a. accept their dying.
   *b. remain free of infection.
   c. experience no bleeding.
   d. have a hematocrit above 35.

10. Your client asks you if he is contaminated now that he is receiving chemotherapy. The best response would be:
    *a. Your urine and bodily secretions will contain the chemotherapy drugs for 24–72 hours after each treatment, so you need to be careful during that time.
    b. Only your blood contains the drugs; you can-not contaminate anyone unless you are actively bleeding.
    c. Once the treatment is finished, you will have no more of the drug in your body.
    d. The drugs will remain in your system for about a month; during that time, you will need to use universal precautions.

11. Your client, who is receiving chemotherapy for breast cancer, tells you that she has noticed ulcers in her mouth. The best response is:
    a. "Stay on a warm liquid diet until the ulcers have healed."
    b. "Your doctor can order a Carafate solution that will help the ulcers heal."
    c. "Gargle with antiseptic solution after each meal to prevent infection."
    *d. "Brush your teeth with baking soda and use a soft toothbrush."

12. Your client is to receive a chemotherapeutic agent known to produce alopecia. He should be instructed to:
    *a. buy a wig before he loses his hair.
    b. get a permanent to give his hair body and prevent hair loss.
    c. brush his hair rigorously to strengthen the roots.
    d. rub his scalp with mineral oils to prevent scalp irritation from hair loss.

13. Alkylating agents act by:
    *a. preventing DNA replication.
    b. preventing RNA replication.
    c. interfering with chromosomal synthesis.
    d. interfering with miosis.

14. Fluorouracil (Adrucil) is active during the follow-ing cell cycle:
    a. G_0 phase
    b. M phase
    *c. S phase
    d. G_2 phase

15. During methotrexate (Amethopterin) therapy, you should assess the client carefully for:
    a. ataxia.
    b. cystitis.
    c. cyanosis.
    *d. jaundice.

16. An indication of a serious reaction to daunoru-bicin (Cerubidin) that should be reported to the physician is:
    a. nausea, vomiting, and diarrhea.
    b. fever and chills.
    c. lethargy, muscle weakness, and depression.
    *d. peripheral edema, tachycardia, and dyspnea.

17. You know your teaching has been effective if your client, who is receiving the hormonal anti-neoplastic agent prednisone (Deltasone), states, "I will take the medication:
    a. on an empty stomach."
    b. about 1 hour after meals."
    *c. with meals."
    d. at bedtime."

18. When a client is receiving hydroxyurea (Hydrea), the following drug may be added to the therapeutic regime to prevent adverse effects:
    a. Hydrochlorothiazide (HydroDIURIL)
    b. Enalapril (Vasotec)
    c. Acetaminophen (Tylenol)
    *d. Allopurinol (Zyloprim)

19. An adverse reaction to vincristine (Oncovin) that you should be assessing for is:
    a. pulmonary fibrosis.
    *b. peripheral neuropathy.
    c. renal failure.
    d. heart failure.

CRITICAL THINKING CASE STUDY

1. It is common to use several drugs to attack a cancer at various places in the cell cycle. Fluorouracil causes hair loss and stomatitis. Mrs. J. should make arrangements for a wig prior to losing her hair. Bone marrow depression commonly occurs, so lab values need to be monitored. An adequate fluid intake will help minimize hemorrhagic cystitis that results from Cytoxan administration.

2. Allow her to express her feelings about her body image change. Ask her if she would like to speak with a cancer survivor.

3. Cytoxan can cause hemorrhagic cystitis. Contact her physician and force fluids.

4. These symptoms can be indicative of heart failure. The physician should be contacted immediately.

65
Drugs Used in Ophthalmic Conditions

MAJOR TOPICS

Structures of the eye
Ophthalmic disorders
Types of ophthalmic drugs

DRUG LIST

Glycerin (Osmoglyn)
Timolol (Timoptic)
Tropicamide (Mydriacyl)

OBJECTIVES

1. Review characteristics of ocular structures that influence drug therapy of eye disorders.
2. Discuss autonomic nervous system (ANS), antimicrobial, anti-inflammatory, and selected miscellaneous drugs in relation to their use in ocular disorders.
3. Use correct techniques to administer ophthalmic medications.

4. Assess for ocular effects of systemic drugs and systemic effects of ophthalmic drugs.
5. Teach clients, family members, or caregivers correct administration of eye medications.
6. For a client with an eye disorder, teach about the importance of taking medications as prescribed to protect and preserve eyesight.

TEACHING STRATEGIES

Classroom

1. Lecture/discussion, using the objectives as an outline.
2. Discuss unique features of administering and observing the effects of ophthalmic medications.
3. Discuss drug therapy of a client with glaucoma, cataract surgery, or eye infection and the subsequent nursing process implications.
4. Discuss the review and application exercises (text, p. 850).
5. Assign small groups to discuss the Critical Thinking Case Study (SG, p. 242).

Clinical Laboratory

1. For clients receiving eye medications, have students verbalize the correct technique(s), administer the drug(s), and observe for systemic effects (e.g., bradycardia with beta blockers).
2. Have students teach clients self-administration of eye drops and ointments.
3. Have students participate in vision screening in health fairs or schools.

TESTBANK QUESTIONS

1. Your client is to begin treatment with pilocarpine. You should instruct her that she may experience:
   a. scleral edema.
   b. a change in the color of her iris.
   c. excessive tearing.
   *d. burning and itching.

2. When assessing a client who is receiving pilocarpine, you will find:
   a. asymmetrically shaped pupils.
   *b. constricted pupils.
   c. dilated pupils.
   d. rapid accommodation.

3. The following statement by your client, who is receiving pilocarpine, leads you to believe that he has understood your teaching:
   a. "A stinging sensation indicates that the medication is lowering my intraocular pressure."
   *b. "My visual acuity will be reduced so I will not drive at night."
   c. "I can expect dryness of my mouth and throat."
   d. "My eyelids should be massaged after administration of the eye drops."

4. Your client is to switch from pilocarpine to timo-lol maleate (Timoptic). Prior to administering the medication, you should check to see if he has a history of:
   a. peripheral vascular disease.
   b. sulfur allergy.
   *c. chronic pulmonary disease.
   d. peptic ulcer disease.

5. Fluorescein (Ful-Glo) can be used in the eye to:
   a. treat conjunctivitis.
   *b. diagnose lesions of the eye.
   c. eliminate pain when a foreign object is removed from the eye.
   d. stain the eye a red color 30 minutes prior to examination.

6. Prednisolone sodium phosphate (Inflamase) is used primarily for:
   a. treatment of fungal eye infections.
   b. management of acute systemic infections that affect vision.
   c. long-term treatment of increased intraocular pressure.
   *d. reduction of scarring and to prevent loss of vision.

7. Acetazolamide (Diamox) works to lower intraocular pressure by:
   a. producing systemic alkalosis.
   *b. interfering with carbonic acid production.
   c. osmotic diuresis.
   d. contraction of ciliary muscles.

CRITICAL THINKING CASE STUDY

1. Pilocarpine is a cholinergic agent that increases the outflow of aqueous humor. Timoptic is a beta-adrenergic blocker that decreases the production of aqueous humor and thereby decreases intraocular pressure.

2. It is important that you take the drops at the prescribed times. Failure to take the medication can jeopardize your vision. Your night vision will be affected; it is not advisable to drive after dark. You should avoid any medication that will increase your intraocular pressure. Make sure that you make all of your health care providers aware that you have glaucoma.

3. You will need to use the medication the rest of your life.

4. Glaucoma is hereditary, but if it is caught early damage can be prevented. Your children should be screened yearly.

66 Drugs Used in Dermatologic Conditions

MAJOR TOPICS
Functions of skin and mucous membranes
Skin disorders
Types of dermatologic drugs

DRUG LIST
Acyclovir (Zovirax)
Benzoyl peroxide (Oxy 5, Panoxyl)
Chlorhexidine (Hibiclens)
Hydrocortisone (Cortril, others)
Hydrogen peroxide
Povidone-iodine (Betadine)

OBJECTIVES

1. Review characteristics of skin structures that influence drug therapy of dermatologic disorders.
2. Discuss antimicrobial, anti-inflammatory, and selected miscellaneous drugs in relation to their use in dermatologic disorders.
3. Use correct techniques to administer dermatologic medications.
4. Teach clients, family members, or caregivers correct administration of dermatologic medications.
5. For clients with "open lesion" skin disorders, teach about the importance and techniques of preventing infection.
6. Practice and teach measures to protect skin from the damaging effects of sun exposure.

TEACHING STRATEGIES

Classroom

1. Lecture/discussion, using the objectives as an outline.
2. Discuss unique features of administering dermatologic medications.
3. Discuss drug therapy of a client with a skin disorder, such as acne or dermatitis, and the associated nursing process implications.
4. Discuss the review and application exercises (text, p. 866).
5. Assign small groups to discuss the Critical Thinking Case Study (SG, p. 245).

Clinical Laboratory

1. Have students assess clients (especially hospitalized or home care clients whose activities are restricted) for skin disorders such as pressure ulcers.
2. For clients receiving dermatologic medications, have students verbalize the correct technique(s), administer the drug(s), and observe responses.

3. Have students teach clients how to apply dermatologic drugs.

4. Have students participate in teaching adolescent groups the facts and myths associated with acne.

5. Have students teach caregivers of elderly clients the importance of preventing pressure ulcers.

TESTBANK QUESTIONS

1. The physician has ordered silver sulfadiazine (Silvadene) for your client's infected burn wound. She asks you why her physician ordered this. The best reply would be:
   *a. "This medication exerts antibacterial action against *Pseudomonas* and other organisms that infect wounds."
   b. "That is an excellent cleaning agent; it will dissolve necrotic materials."
   c. "Drug resistance can develop from other agents, so this medication is better."
   d. "When the skin is broken, more of the drug is absorbed systemically, so this preparation is more effective than oral agents."

2. An effective topical agent for acne is:
   a. acetic acid.
   *b. benzoyl peroxide.
   c. chlorhexidine (Hibiclens).
   d. pHisoHex.

3. A client with *Candida* infection is to use a dilute solution of acetic acid as a douche. What instruction will you give her?
   a. "Open lesions can occur with chronic use of acetic acid douches."
   b. "Acetic acid douches are very drying to the mucous membranes and can interfere with pregnancy."
   *c. "Acetic acid solution administered as a douche should help your burning and itching."
   d. "Prolonged use of acetic acid as a douche can cause you to develop cutaneous dermatophytosis."

4. The physician orders haloprogin (Halotex) for your client's initial outbreak of tinea pedis. Which of the following instructions should you give her?
   a. "Apply topically to the lesions 6 times a day for 7 days."
   *b. "Wash your feet before each application and use it in the morning and at bedtime for 2–4 weeks."
   c. "You should leave the medication on for an hour, then remove it with soap and water."
   d. "Apply the medication no more than once a day. Overuse will cause severe inflammation."

5. Your client's physician prescribes triamcinolone acetonide (Aristocort) for dermatitis. An adverse effect of excessive administration of this medication is:
   *a. atrophy of the skin.
   b. superinfection.
   c. hypervitaminosis.
   d. loss of pigmentation in the area of the application.

6. The drug of choice for treating oral candidiasis is:
   *a. nystatin (Mycostatin).
   b. acetic acid.
   c. acrisorcin (Akrinol).
   d. zinc oxide.

7. Which of the following medications would be most helpful to relieve the itching of chicken pox?
   a. Coal tar (Balnetar)
   *b. Colloidal oatmeal (Aveeno)
   c. Trioxsalen (Trisoralen)
   d. Sutilains (Travase)

8. Which of the following instructions should be given to a client using tretinoin (Retin-A)?
   a. "Avoid green leafy vegetables."
   b. "Drink lots of fluids that are high in vitamin C."
   *c. "Avoid excessive exposure to sunlight."
   d. "Apply the medication at night."

9. Your client asks you what the cause of acne is. The best reply would be:
   *a. "Acne is caused by excessive production of sebum and obstruction of hair follicles. Wash your face 3 times a day to keep it clean."
   b. "Emotional stress can cause acne; try and relax."
   c. "You must be eating too much fat; avoid peanut butter and chocolate."
   d. "Acne is hereditary, but you will outgrow it; so be patient."

10. Your neighbor calls you and asks you what ingredient would help her psoriasis. You should recommend a product containing:
    a. benzoyl peroxide.
    b. hydrogen peroxide.
    *c. coal tar.
    d. acetic acid.

11. An agent used to remove warts, corns, or calluses is called a:
    a. demelanizing agent.
    b. enzyme agent.
    *c. keratolytic agent.
    d. melanizing agent.

12. Which of the following statements is true regarding topical preparations? Absorption is increased when:
    a. the outermost layer of the dermis is dehydrated.
    b. the skin is intact.
    c. the medication is applied to the palms of hands and soles of feet.
    *d. drugs are left in place for long periods of time.

13. The following is *not* a property of medications applied topically:
    a. Anesthetic
    b. Anti-inflammatory
    c. Bacteriostatic
    *d. Antiarrhythmic

CRITICAL THINKING CASE STUDY

1. Wash your face gently and apply the medication topically once a day. It is an irritant so your face will appear red.

2. Emotional stress and birth control pills can aggravate acne. Talk to your physician about changing your medication.

3. Instruct her to stop using the medication and apply clean, cold compresses to her face until it has healed.

4. Discuss with her why she medicated 4 times per day. Ask her if she has any symptoms of hypervitaminosis A: nausea, vomiting, headache, blurred vision, eye irritation, or muscle skeletal pain.

67
Drug Use During Pregnancy and Lactation

MAJOR TOPICS

Maternal-placental-fetal circulation
Maternal changes of pregnancy
Drug effects during pregnancy
Fetal therapeutics
Management of pregnancy-induced symptoms
Management of chronic diseases during pregnancy
Neonatal therapeutics
Drugs used during labor, delivery, and lactation

DRUG LIST

Carboprost (Hemabate)
Oxytocin (Pitocin)
Ritodrine (Yutopar)
Terbutaline (Brethine)

OBJECTIVES

1. Discuss reasons for avoiding or minimizing drug therapy during pregnancy and lactation.
2. Describe selected teratogenic drugs.
3. Disease guidelines for drug therapy of pregnancy-induced signs and symptoms.
4. Discuss guidelines for drug therapy of chronic disorders during pregnancy and lactation.
5. Teach adolescents and young adult women to avoid prescribed and OTC drugs when possible and to inform physicians and dentists if there is a possibility of pregnancy.

6. Discuss drugs used during labor and delivery in terms of their effects on mother and newborn infant.
7. Describe abortifacients in terms of characteristics and nursing process implications.

TEACHING STRATEGIES

Classroom

1. If there is a separate pharmacology course, review the course syllabus and talk with the instructor of obstetric nursing regarding drug-related content to promote needed coverage and avoid unnecessary repetition.

2. Discuss hazards of taking any drugs, smoking cigarettes, or drinking alcohol during pregnancy or if sexually active and not using effective contraception.

3. Emphasize the nursing role in teaching pregnant women nondrug-related interventions to relieve pregnancy-induced symptoms.

4. Discuss or have students write answers to the review and application exercises (text, p. 886).

5. Discuss the Critical Thinking Case Study (SG, p. 249).

6. Ask students to share their opinions and attitudes about abortion and the nurse's role in caring for clients undergoing abortion.

Clinical Laboratory

1. Have students teach adolescent and adult females of reproductive potential regarding desirability of avoiding drugs, including OTC preparations, when there is any chance of becoming pregnant.

2. Have students assist with prenatal assessment, monitoring, and teaching in an obstetric clinic or physician's office.

3. For a group of prenatal clients, have students list the drugs being taken and evaluate their teratogenic potential.

4. Assign students to prepare a nursing care plan or write a short paper about drug therapy for pregnant clients with chronic diseases, such as asthma, diabetes mellitus, epilepsy, or hypertension.

TESTBANK QUESTIONS

1. After receiving magnesium sulfate, your client develops magnesium toxicity. You should administer:
   a. oxygen.
   b. epinephrine.
   c. potassium chloride.
   *d. calcium gluconate.

2. The infant of a mother who received magnesium sulfate during labor should be monitored for:
   a. tachypnea.
   b. paralytic ileus.
   c. dysrhythmias.
   *d. neuromuscular depression.

3. During labor, your client requests pain medication. You know that pain medication will:
   a. reduce signs of fetal distress.
   b. promote fetal hyperactivity.
   *c. prolong the latent stage of labor.
   d. increase uterine contractions.

4. Your client exhibits hypotension related to epidural anesthesia. You should administer:
   *a. oxygen and place the client in left lateral position.
   b. meperidine (Demerol) and place the client in semi-Fowler's position.
   c. pitocin (Oxytocin) and place the client in Trendelenburg position.
   d. a normal saline bolus and place the client in a supine position.

5. An insulin dependent diabetic may require an increased insulin dose during pregnancy due to the presence of:
   *a. HPL.
   b. prolactin.
   c. oxytocin.
   d. progesterone.

6. To stop premature labor, the following drug may be administered:
   a. Calcium carbonate
   *b. Terbutaline (Brethine)
   c. Diazepam (Valium)
   d. Dinoprostone (Prostin E)

7. Oxytocin is contraindicated if the client has:
   a. multiple sclerosis.
   b. renal disease.
   c. hypertension,
   *d. placenta previa.

CRITICAL THINKING CASE STUDY

1. The suppository will "ripen" your cervix causing it to dilate more easily, and the oxytocin will induce contractions.

2. Evaluate her pain. Help her to use her Lamaze breathing. Discuss with her the implications for labor if she receives pain medication.

3. Stop the administration of the pain medication and immediately check her vital signs. If her blood pressure has dropped, place her on her side and administer O_2. Check the fetal heart rate, and then contact the physician STAT.

APPENDIX A
DRUG JEOPARDY

DRUG JEOPARDY GUIDELINES

Supplies Needed

1. Drug Jeopardy overhead transparencies (masters provided for three games).

2. Overhead projector.

3. Several thousand dollars of play money (can be cut from green construction paper and labeled in $100, $500, and $1,000 denominations).

4. Post-it notes, cut into squares, to cover the money category on the Drug Jeopardy transparency, once that category has been used.

Playing

1. Divide students into small groups (two to five students per group) in clinical or classroom settings.

2. Give each group several thousand dollars of play money; same amount to each group.

3. Designate a student "banker" (request a volunteer or choose one) and give him or her several thousand dollars of play money.

4. Place transparency on projector, showing headings and money columns.

5. Ask a group to choose a category and amount (e.g., Antidotes for $100).

6. Read the statement prepared for that heading and dollar amount.

7. The "working" group can consult among its members and give an answer in question form. If the question corresponds to the prepared question, the banker pays the group $100. If the group answers incorrectly, it pays the banker $100. If the group feels unable to answer, ask the next group if it wants to try.

8. Cover the appropriate category so everyone can see it has been used and is no longer available.

9. Continue until all categories are used or stop at any time.

10. The group with the most money is the winner.

(This game can be used in a pharmacology class, in a clinical postconference, and with graduating seniors as an NCLEX review exercise.)

Alternate Method

Another way to play Drug Jeopardy is to let each row of students take turns responding, without keeping score or using money. This method takes less time, but also decreases the competitive and collaborative aspects.

DRUG JEOPARDY: ANTIMICROBIAL DRUGS

Penicillins	Cephalo-sporins	Amino-glycosides	Tetra-cyclines	Miscellaneous Anti-infectives
$100	$100	$100	$100	$100
$200	$200	$200	$200	$200
$300	$300	$300	$300	$300
$400	$400	$400	$400	$400
$500	$500	$500	$500	$500

		Statement (Instructor) "The answer is..."	**Question (Students)** "What is/are..."
Category:	**PENICILLINS**		
	$100	The first penicillin to be introduced.	penicillin G?
	$200	Penicillins are rapidly excreted by this organ.	the kidney?
	$300	This broad spectrum semisynthetic penicillin is bactericidal.	ampicillin?
	$400	This preparation contains amoxicillin and potassium clavulanate.	Augmentin?
	$500	This drug when given concurrently with penicillin will increase its serum drug levels.	probenecid (Benemid)?
Category:	**CEPHALOSPORINS**		
	$100	This drug penetrates the cerebral spinal fluid in the presence of inflamed meninges.	cefuroxime?
	$200	Prototype of 1st-generation cephalosporins.	cephalothin (Keflin)?
	$300	The 3rd generation cephalosporin first approved for once a day dosing.	ceftriaxone (Rocephin)?
	$400	The only cephalosporin that does not need to be reduced in renal failure.	cefoperazone (Cefobid)?
	$500	The antibiotic that when administered with cephalosporins will decrease their effect.	tetracycline?
Category:	**AMINOGLYCOSIDES**		
	$100	Aminoglycosides have two major side effects.	nephrotoxicity and ototoxicity?
	$200	The aminoglycoside commonly used preoperatively to decrease bacterial flora in the colon.	neomycin?
	$300	The first aminoglycoside developed.	streptomycin?
	$400	Maintenance doses of aminoglycosides are based on the following levels.	the peaks and troughs of serum drug levels?
	$500	This drug, when administered concurrently with aminoglycosides, increases the risk of nephrotoxicity.	tetracycline?

	Statement (Instructor) "The answer is..."	**Question (Students)** "What is/are..."

Category: TETRACYCLINES

$100	A highly lipid-soluble tetracycline that reaches therapeutic levels in CSF.	doxycycline (Vibramycin)?
$200	A group in which the use of tetracycline is contraindicated.	pregnant women or preschool-age children?
$300	Tetracycline most likely to cause photosensitivity.	demeclocycline (Declomycin)?
$400	Probably the most frequently used tetracycline.	tetracycline (Achromycin)?
$500	The only tetracycline considered safe in clients with renal impairment.	doxycycline (Vibramycin)?

Category: MISCELLANEOUS ANTI-INFECTIVES

$100	A drug that is similar in activity against gram-negative bacteria to aminoglycosides but does not cause kidney damage and hearing loss.	aztreonam (Azactam)?
$200	This medication is used to treat pseudomembranous colitis.	vancomycin (Vancocin)?
$300	When this drug is initiated, clients need a CBC, platelet count, reticulocyte count, and serum iron every 3 days.	chloramphenicol (Chloromycetin)?
$400	An adverse effect of the administration of chloramphenicol (Chloromycetin)	blood dyscrasias?
$500	Nephrotoxicity is an adverse effect of the administration of this drug.	vancomycin (Vancocin)?

DRUG JEOPARDY: ANS DRUGS

Indications for Use	ANS Receptors	Nursing Process	Adverse Drug Reactions	Miscel- laneous
$100	$100	$100	$100	$100
$200	$200	$200	$200	$200
$300	$300	$300	$300	$300
$400	$400	$400	$400	$400
$500	$500	$500	$500	$500

		Statement (Instructor) "The answer is..."	Question (Students) "What is/are..."
Category:	**INDICATIONS FOR USE**		
	$100	Asthma and lung problems.	adrenergics?
	$200	Hypertension.	beta blockers or alpha blockers?
	$300	The type of beta blocker recommended for asthmatics and diabetics.	cardioselective beta blockers?
	$400	Myasthenia gravis.	cholinergics?
	$500	Bradycardia.	atropine?
Category:	**ANS RECEPTORS**		
	$100	Stimulation of $beta_1$ receptors.	cardiac stimulation or increased rate and force of myocardial contraction?
	$200	Stimulation of $beta_2$ receptors.	bronchodilation?
	$300	Stimulation of cholinergic receptors.	muscle contraction?
	$400	Blockage of beta receptors.	decreased heart rate and force of myocardial contraction? decreased blood pressure? bronchoconstriction? bradycardia?
	$500	Stimulation of $alpha_1$ receptors.	vasoconstriction?
Category:	**NURSING PROCESS**		
	$100	Assess heart rate and blood pressure for decrease.	effects of beta blockers?
	$200	Assess heart rate for increase.	anticholinergics or atropine?
	$300	Teach clients not to stop these drugs abruptly.	beta blockers?
	$400	Knowledge deficit: drug usage and effects.	a nursing diagnosis that indicates a need for client teaching?
	$500	Teach clients to increase intake of high-fiber foods to decrease constipation.	drugs with anticholinergic effects?

Category: **ADVERSE DRUG REACTIONS**

$100	Dry mouth, tachycardia, urinary retention, constipation, and blurred vision.	adverse effects of anticholinergic drugs (or atropine)?
$200	Drugs in this group cause anticholinergic effects.	adverse effects of antipsychotics (or antidepressants or antihistamines)?
$300	Cardiac arrhythmias and hypertension.	adverse effects of adrenergic drugs?
$400	Bradycardia, congestive heart failure (CHF).	adverse effects of beta blockers?
$500	Bronchoconstriction.	adverse effects of nonselective beta blockers (also cholinergic drugs)?

Category: **MISCELLANEOUS**

$100	A drug that blocks both $beta_1$ and $beta_2$ receptors.	propranolol (Inderal)?
$200	A drug that stimulates both alpha and beta receptors.	epinephrine?
$300	A drug that blocks the action of acetylcholine.	atropine?
$400	Drugs that decrease nasal congestion by causing vasoconstriction in nasal mucosa.	adrenergics?
$500	OTC drugs to be avoided or used very cautiously by people with hypertension, angina pectoris, or tachyarrhythmias.	adrenergics (or cold and asthma remedies?)

DRUG JEOPARDY: CARDIOVASCULAR DRUGS

Indications for Use	Adverse Effects	Drug Interactions	Nursing Process	Miscellaneous
$100	$100	$100	$100	$100
$200	$200	$200	$200	$200
$300	$300	$300	$300	$300
$400	$400	$400	$400	$400
$500	$500	$500	$500	$500

STATEMENTS AND QUESTIONS: CARDIOVASCULAR DRUGS

	Statement (Instructor) "The answer is..."	Question (Students) "What is/are..."
Category: INDICATIONS FOR USE		
$100	A drug used for CHF and atrial fibrillation.	digoxin (Lanoxin)?
$200	A drug group used to decrease fluid retention and edema.	diuretics?
$300	Drugs used to lower serum cholesterol.	lovastatin (Mevacor) and related drugs?
$400	Alpha$_1$-receptor blocking agents used to treat hypertension.	doxazosin (Cardura) and related drugs?
$500	Two drug groups used for both angina and hypertension.	beta blockers and calcium channel blockers?
Category: ADVERSE EFFECTS		
$100	Hypokalemia.	an adverse effect of diuretics?
$200	Hypotension.	an adverse effect of antihypertensive (and antiarrhythmic) drugs?
$300	Bleeding.	an adverse effect of anticoagulant, antiplatelet, and thrombolytic drugs?
$400	Arrhythmias.	an adverse effect of digoxin (Lanoxin)?
$500	Hepatotoxicity	an adverse effect of lovastatin (Mevacor) and related drugs?
Category: DRUG INTERACTIONS		
$100	Drugs that decrease absorption of digoxin.	antacids?
$200	Drugs that increase effects of digoxin.	quinidine, nifedipine, verapamil?
$300	A drug to reverse diuretic-induced hypokalemia.	potassium chloride?
$400	A drug to reverse digoxin- or beta blocker-induced bradycardia.	atropine
$500	OTC drugs that may decrease effects of antihypertensive drugs.	nasal decongestants and appetite suppressants (adrenergic drugs)?

		Statement (Instructor) "The answer is..."	Question (Students) "What is/are..."

Category: **NURSING PROCESS**

	Statement (Instructor)	Question (Students)
$100	Cardiovascular drugs with which blood pressure should be monitored.	antihypertensives, antianginals, and antiarrhythmics?
$200	Cardiovascular drugs with which pulse should be monitored.	digoxin and beta blockers?
$300	Drugs with which clients must be assessed for signs and symptoms of bleeding.	anticoagulants, antiplatelet agents, and thrombolytics.
$400	A drug with which serum drug levels should be monitored.	digoxin (Lanoxin)?
$500	Drugs with which serum electrolytes should be monitored.	digoxin and diuretics?

Category: **MISCELLANEOUS**

$100	The antidote for an overdose of warfarin (Coumadin).	vitamin K?
$200	The antidote for an overdose of heparin.	protamine sulfate?
$300	The usual daily maintenance dose of digoxin.	0.125–0.25 mg?
$400	The acceptable range of serum potassium levels.	3.5–5.0 mEq/L?
$500	A drug group used to treat both hypertension and congestive heart failure.	angiotensin-converting enzyme (ACE) inhibitors?

APPENDIX B
TRANSPARENCY MASTERS

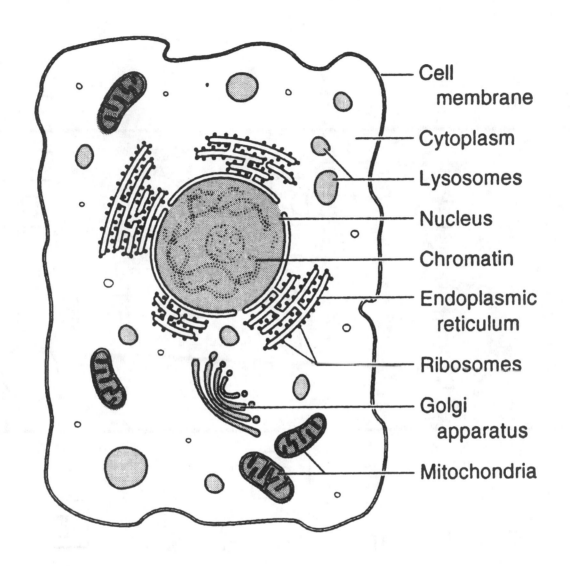

Cell membrane

Cytoplasm

Lysosomes

Nucleus

Chromatin

Endoplasmic reticulum

Ribosomes

Golgi apparatus

Mitochondria

Blood
Stream

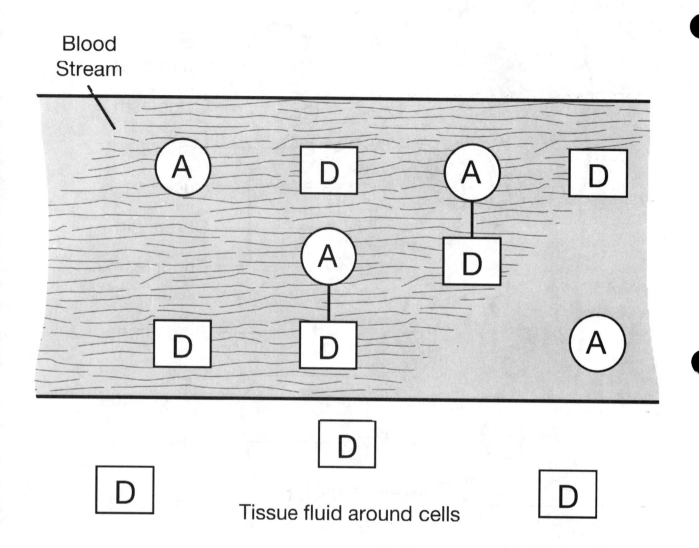

Tissue fluid around cells

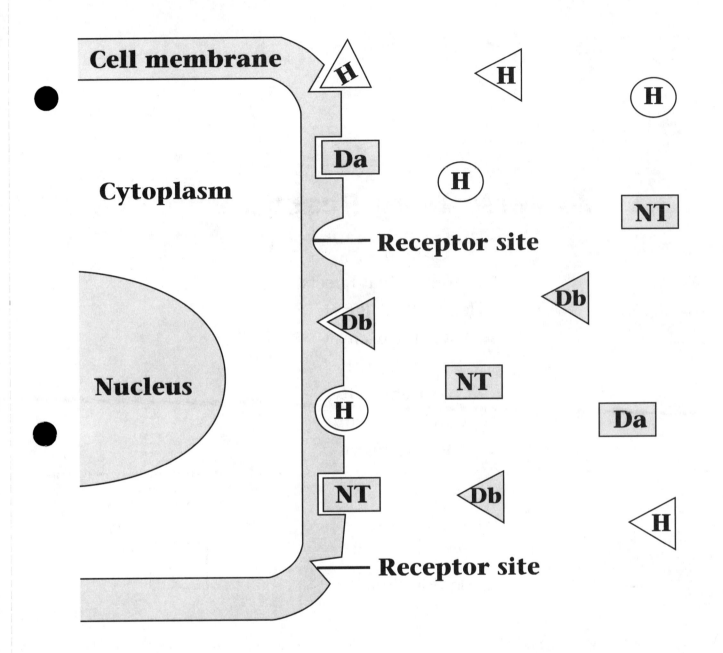

Cell membrane

Cytoplasm

Nucleus

Receptor site

Receptor site

Adverse Drug Reactions

CNS Effects
Gastrointestinal Effects
Hematologic Effects
Hepatotoxicity
Nephrotoxicity
Hypersensitivity
Carcinogenicity
Teratogenicity

Chapter 2

Five Rights of Drug Administration

Right Drug

- Interpret physician's orders accurately
- Question the order if the name of the drug is not clear or if the drug seems inappropriate for the client's condition
- Read drug labels accurately

Right Route

- Use correct techniques for all routes of administration
- Always use appropriate landmarks to identify IM injection sites
- For IV medications, follow authoritative instructions for preparation and administration

Right Time

- Schedule to maximize therapeutic effects and minimize adverse effects
- Omit or delay doses when indicated by the client's condition

Right Dose

- Interpret abbreviations accurately
- Interpret measurements accurately
- Calculate dosages accurately

Right Client

- Check name bands on institutionalized clients
- Verify name on ambulatory clients

BOX 4-1. MEDICATION HISTORY

Name _____ Age _____

Health problems, acute and chronic

Are you allergic to any medications?

If yes, describe specific effects or symptoms.

PART 1: PRESCRIPTION MEDICATIONS

1. Do you take any prescription medications on a regular basis?

2. If yes, ask the following about each medication.

    Name   Dose

    Frequency   Specific times

    How long taken   Reason

3. Are you able to take this medicine as prescribed?

4. Does anyone else help you take your medications?

5. What information or instructions were you given when the medications were first prescribed?

6. Do you think the medication is doing what it was prescribed to do?

7. Have you had any problems that you attribute to the medication?

8. Do you take any prescription medications on an irregular basis? If yes, ask the following about each medication.

    Name   Reason

    Dose   How long taken

    Frequency

PART 2: NONPRESCRIPTION MEDICATIONS

Do you take OTC medications?

		Medication		
Problem	Yes/No	Name	Amount	Frequency
Pain				
Headache				
Sleep				
Cold				
Indigestion				
Heartburn				
Diarrhea				
Constipation				
Other				

PART 3: SOCIAL DRUGS

	Yes/No	Amount
Coffee		
Tea		
Cola drinks		
Alcohol		
Tobacco		

Chapter 4

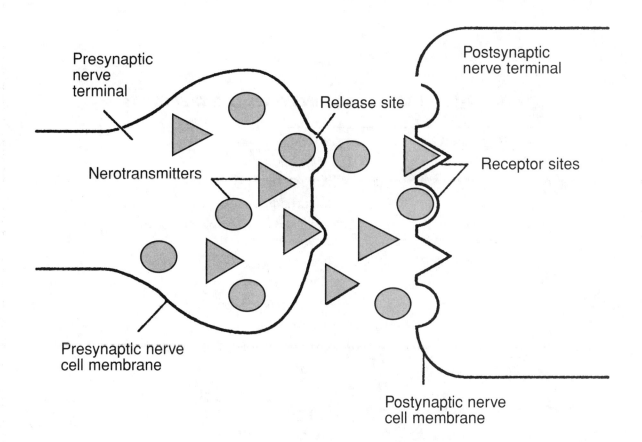

Presynaptic
nerve
terminal

Release site

Postsynaptic
nerve terminal

Nerotransmitters

Receptor sites

Presynaptic nerve
cell membrane

Postynaptic nerve
cell membrane

TABLE 7-1. PROSTAGLANDINS AND THEIR EFFECTS

Prostaglandin	Effect
D_2	Bronchoconstriction
E_2	Vasodilation
	Bronchodilation
	Increased activity of gastrointestinal (GI) smooth muscle
	Increased sensitivity to pain
	Increased body temperature
F_2	Bronchoconstriction
	Increased uterine contraction
	Increased activity of GI smooth muscle
I_2 (prostacyclin)	Vasodilation
	Decreased platelet aggregation
Tnromboxane A_2	Vasoconstriction
	Increased platelet aggregation

Chapter 7

TABLE 7-2. CLINICAL INDICATIONS FOR COMMONLY USED ANALGESIC–ANTIPYRETIC–ANTI-INFLAMMATORY DRUGS

Generic/Trade Name	Pain	Fever	Osteoarthritis	Rheumatoid Arthritis	Juvenile Rheumatoid Arthritis	Dysmenorrhea	Acute Painful Shoulder	Ankylosing Spondylitis	Bursitis	Gout	Tendinitis
Acetaminophen (Tylenol, others)	✓	✓									
Acetylsalicylic Acid (Aspirin)	✓	✓	✓	✓	✓	✓	✓	✓	✓	✓	✓
Diclofenac (Voltaren)			✓	✓				✓			
Diflunisal (Dolobid)	✓		✓	✓							
Etodolac (Lodine)	✓		✓								
Fenoprofen (Nalfon)	✓		✓	✓							
Flurbiprofen (Ansaid)			✓	✓							
Ibuprofen (Motrin, others)	✓	✓	✓	✓		✓				✓	✓
Indomethacin (Indocin)			✓	✓			✓	✓	✓	✓	✓
Ketoprofen (Orudis)	✓		✓	✓		✓			✓	✓	✓
Ketorolac (Toradol)	✓										
Nabumetone (Relafen)			✓	✓							
Naproxen (Naprosyn)	✓		✓	✓	✓	✓		✓	✓	✓	✓
Oxaprozin (Daypro)			✓	✓							
Piroxicam (Feldene)			✓	✓							
Sulindac (Clinoril)			✓	✓			✓	✓	✓	✓	✓
Tolmetin (Tolectin)			✓	✓	✓						

Antianxiety Benzodiazepines

Generic Name	Trade Name
Alprazolam	Xanax
Chlordiazepoxide	Librium
Clonazepam	Klonopin
Clorazepate	Tranxene
Diazepam	Valium
Halazepam	Paxipam
Lorazepam	Ativan
Midazolam	Versed
Oxazepam	Serax
Prazepam	Centrax

Chapter 8

Hypnotic Benzodiazepines

Generic Name	Trade Name
Estazolam	ProSom
Flurazepam	Dalmane
Quazepam	Doral
Temazepam	Restoril
Triazolam	Halcion

Types of Antidepressants

Tricyclic Antidepressants (TCAs)

Monoamine Oxidase Inhibitors (MAO Inhibitors or MAOI)

Selective Serotonin Reuptake Inhibitors (SSRI)

Miscellaneous or Heterocyclic

Table 17-1. Adrenergic Receptors

Type	Location	Effects of Stimulation
Alpha$_1$	Blood vessels	Vasoconstriction
	Gastrointestinal (GI) tract	Inhibition
	Uterus	Contraction
	Eye	Blinking, mydriasis
Alpha$_2$	Presynaptic adrenergic nerve endings	Inhibits release of norepinephrine
	Platelets	Aggregation
Beta$_1$	Heart	Increased heart rate, force of contraction, automaticity, and rate of AV conduction
	Adipose tissue	Lipolysis
Beta$_2$	Bronchioles	Bronchodilation
	Arterioles of skeletal muscle	Vasodilation
	GI tract	Decreased motility and tone
	Liver	Glycogenolysis, gluconeo-genesis
	Urinary bladder	Relaxed detrusor muscle
	Pregnant uterus	Relaxation

Effects of Beta Blockers

1. Decreased force of myocardial contraction
2. Decreased cardiac output
3. Decreased blood pressure
4. Decreased heart rate
5. Decreased automaticity of ectopic pacemakers
6. Slowed conduction through the AV node
7. Less effective metabolism of glucose
8. Less ability to respond to stress
9. Less ability to increase heart rate and cardiac output in response to exercise or activity

Common Adverse Effects

1. Bradycardia
2. Congestive heart failure
3. Weakness, fatigue
4. Bronchoconstriction

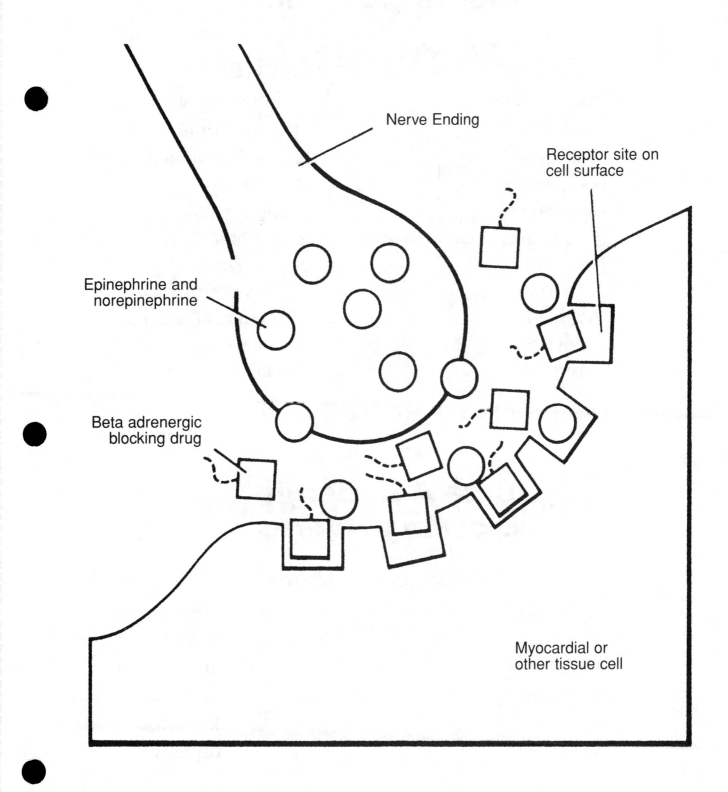

Nerve Ending

Receptor site on
cell surface

Epinephrine and
norepinephrine

Beta adrenergic
blocking drug

Myocardial or
other tissue cell

Chapter 19

Beta Adrenergic Blocking Agents

Nonselective Drugs

Generic Name	Trade Name
Carteolol	Cartrol, Ocupress
Labetalol*	Trandate, Normodyne
Levobunolol	Betagan
Metipranolol	Optipranolol
Nadolol	Corgard
Penbutolol	Levatol
Pindolol	Visken
Propranolol	Inderal
Sotalol	Betapace
Timolol	Blocadren, Timoptic

* Labetalol is also an alpha-adrenergic blocking agent

Beta Adrenergic Blocking Agents

Cardioselective Drugs

Acebutolol	Sectral
Atenolol	Tenormin
Betaxolol	Betoptic, Kerlone
Bisoprolol	Zebeta
Esmolol	Brevibloc
Metoprolol	Lopressor

Beta Adrenergic Blocking Agents

Cardiovascular Indications for Use

	Angina Pectoris	Hyper-tension	Tachy-arrhythmias	Myocardial Infarction
Acebutolol (Sectral)		X	X	
Atenolol (Tenormin)	X	X		X
Betaxolol* (Kerlone)		X		
Bisoprolol (Zebeta)		X		
Carteolol* (Cartrol)		X		
Esmolol (Brevibloc)			X	
Labetalol (Trandate, Normodyne)		X		
Metoprolol (Lopressor)	X	X		X
Nadolol (Corgard)	X	X		
Penbutolol (Levatol)		X		
Pindolol (Visken)		X		
Propranolol (Inderal)	X	X	X	X
Sotalol (Betapace)			X	
Timolol* (Blocadren)		X		X

*Betaxolol (Betoptic), carteolol (Ocupress), and timolol (Timoptic) are also available in ophthalmic preparations for treatment of glaucoma.

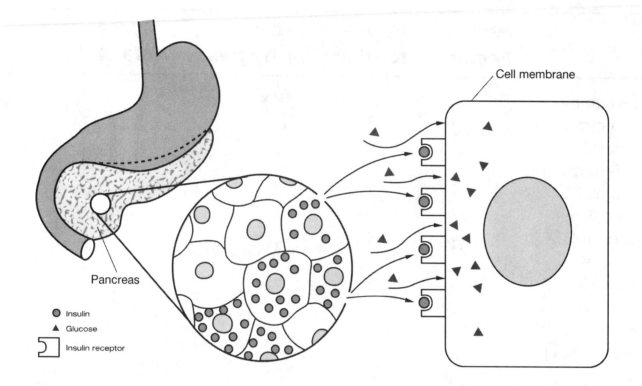

Cell membrane

Pancreas

- ● Insulin
- ▲ Glucose
- ⊐ Insulin receptor

Chapter 27

Beta Lactam Antibiotics

Penicillins
Cephalosporins
Carbapenems
Monobactams

Penicillin Nucleus

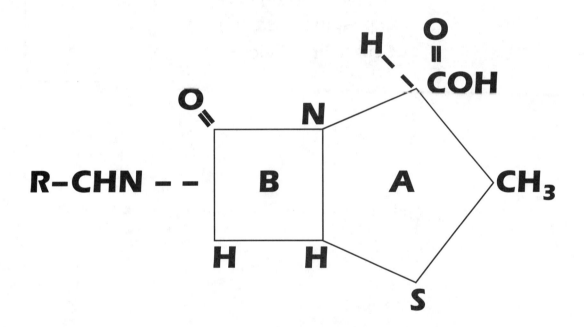

B = Beta Lactam Ring

Cephalosporins

First Generation

Cefadroxil (Duricef)

Cefazolin (Ancef, Kefzol)

Cephalexin (Keflex)

Cephalothin (Keflin)

Cephapirin (Cefadyl)

Cephradine (Velosef)

Chapter 34

Cephalosporins

Second Generation

Cefaclor (Ceclor)

Cefamandole (Mandol)

Cefmetazole (Zefazone)

Cefonicid (Monocid)

Ceforanide (Precef)

Cefotetan (Cefotan)

Cefoxitin (Mefoxin)

Cefprozil (Cefzil)

Cefuroxime (Zinacef)

Loracarbef (Lorabid)

Cephalosporins

Third Generation

Cefixime (Suprax)

Cefoperazone (Cefobid)

Cefpodoxime (Vantin)

Cefotaxime (Claforan)

Ceftazidime (Fortaz)

Ceftibuten (Cedax)

Ceftizoxime (Cefizox)

Ceftriaxone (Rocephin)

Moxalactam (Moxam)

Cephalosporins

Fourth Generation

Cefepime (Maxipime)

Aminoglycosides

Amikacin (Amikin)

Gentamicin (Garamycin)

Netilmicin (Netromycin)

Tobramycin (Nebcin)

Kanamycin (Kantrex)

Neomycin (Mycifradin)

Streptomycin

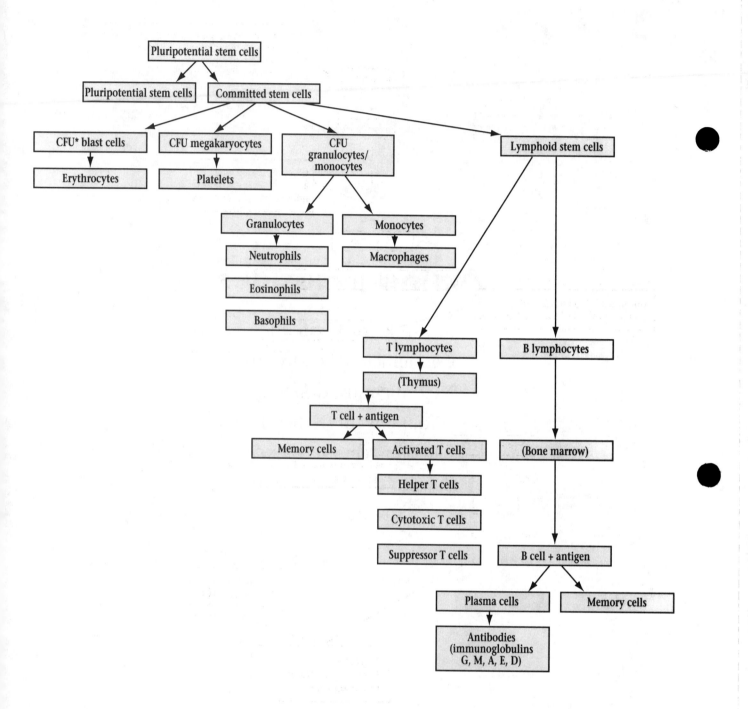

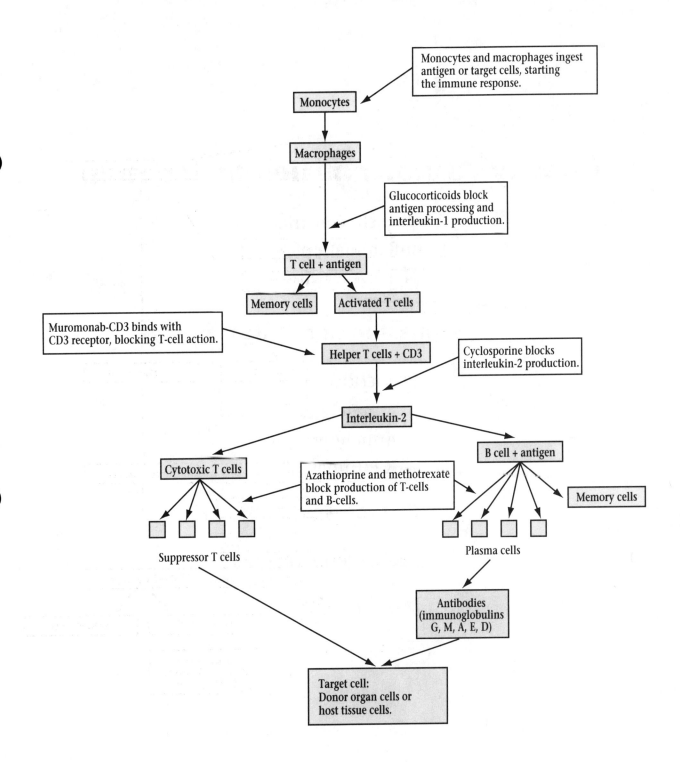

Monocytes and macrophages ingest antigen or target cells, starting the immune response.

Monocytes

Macrophages

Glucocorticoids block antigen processing and interleukin-1 production.

T cell + antigen

Memory cells

Activated T cells

Muromonab-CD3 binds with CD3 receptor, blocking T-cell action.

Helper T cells + CD3

Cyclosporine blocks interleukin-2 production.

Interleukin-2

Cytotoxic T cells

Azathioprine and methotrexate block production of T-cells and B-cells.

B cell + antigen

Memory cells

Suppressor T cells

Plasma cells

Antibodies (immunoglobulins G, M, A, E, D)

Target cell: Donor organ cells or host tissue cells.

Chapter 45

Airway Abnormalities in Asthma

Bronchoconstriction
Inflammation
Hyperreactivity

Antiasthmatic Drugs

Bronchodilators

Adrenergics

Anticholinergics

Xanthines

Corticosteroids

Leukotriene inhibitors

Mast cell stabilizers

Chapter 47

Nonsedating Antihistamines

Astemizole (Hismanal)

Fexofenadine (Allegra)

Loratadine (Claritin)

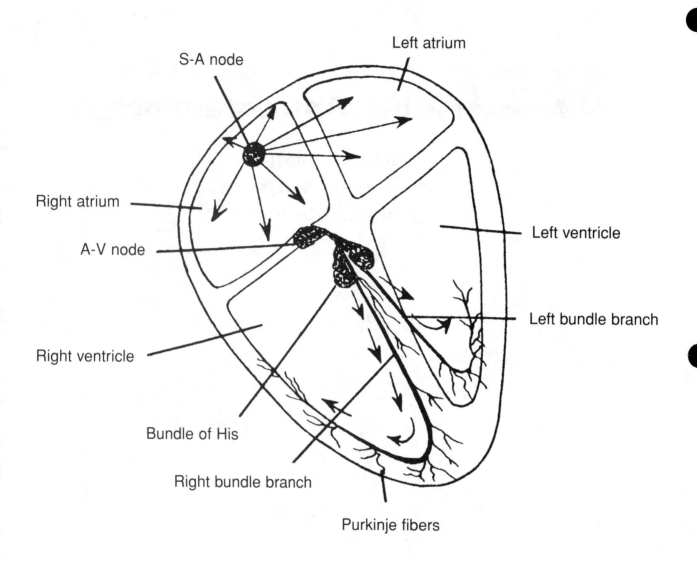

Chapter 48

S-A node

Left atrium

Right atrium

A-V node

Left ventricle

Right ventricle

Left bundle branch

Bundle of His

Right bundle branch

Purkinje fibers

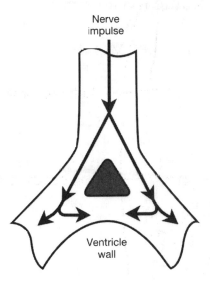

Normal conduction

Nerve impulse

Ventricle wall

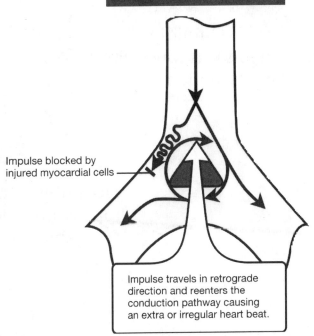

Unidirectional blockage of conduction

Impulse blocked by injured myocardial cells

Impulse travels in retrograde direction and reenters the conduction pathway causing an extra or irregular heart beat.

Antiarrhythmic Drugs

Class I Sodium Channel Blockers (local anesthetics)

IA

Quinidine
Procainamide (Pronestyl, Procan)
Disopyramide (Norpace)

IB

Lidocaine (Xylocaine)
Tocainide (Tonocard)
Mexilitene (Mexitil)

IC

Flecainide (Tambocor)
Propafenone (Rhythmol)
Moricizine* (Ethmozine)

*Moricizine is not classified as IA, IB, or IC, but it has some properties of each group.

Chapter 52

Antiarrhythmic Drugs

Class II Beta Blockers

Acebutolol (Sectral)
Esmolol (Brevibloc)
Propranolol (Inderal)

Class III Potassium Channel Blockers

Amiodarone (Cordarone)
Bretylium (Bretylol)
Sotalol* (Betapace)

Class IV Calcium Channel Blockers

Diltiazem (Cardizem)
Verapamil (Calan, Isoptin)

Unclassified

Adenosine (Adenocard)
Ibutilide (Corvert)
Magnesium sulfate

*Although sotalol is a beta blocker, its antiarrhythmic properties are similar to Class III drugs.

Calcium Channel Blockers

Amlodipine (Norvasc)
Bepridil (Vascor)
Diltiazem (Cardizem)
Felodipine (Plendil)
Isradipine (DynaCirc)
Nicardipine (Cardene)
Nifedipine (Adalat, Procardia)
Nimodipine (Nimotop)
Nisoldipine (Sular)
Verapamil (Calan, Isoptin)

Chapter 53

Muscle relaxation

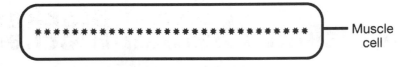

Muscle
cell

A

Muscle contraction

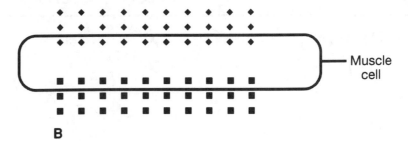

Muscle
cell

B

Calcium-blocking drugs

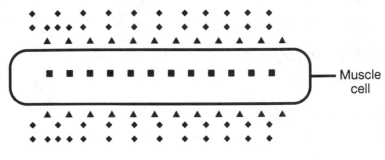

Muscle
cell

C

Calcium Channel Blockers

Cardiovascular Indications for Use

	Angina Pectoris	Hyper-tension	Tachy-arrhythmias
Amlodipine (Norvasc)	X	X	
Bepridil (Vascor)	X		
Diltiazem (Cardizem)	X	X+	
Felodipine (Plendil)		X	
Isradipine (DynaCirc)		X	
Nicardipine (Cardene)	X	X	
Nifedipine (Adalat, Procardia)	X	X+	
Nimodipine (Nimotop)*			
Nisoldipine (Sular)		X	
Verapamil (Calan, Isoptin)	X	X	X

*Nimodipine approved only for treatment of subarachnoid hemorrhage.

+Only the sustained release formulations (diltiazem SR and nifedipine SR) are approved for treatment of hypertension.

Chapter 53

Factors That Regulate Blood Pressure

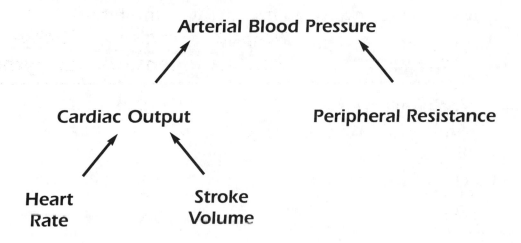

Arterial Blood Pressure

Cardiac Output   Peripheral Resistance

Heart Rate   Stroke Volume

Chapter 55

Antihypertensive Drugs

Angiotensin-Converting Enzyme (ACE) Inhibitors

Angiotensin II Receptor Antagonists

Antiadrenergics

Alpha$_1$ blockers
Alpha$_2$ agonists
Beta blockers

Calcium Channel Blockers

Diuretics

Vasodilators (direct-acting)

Chapter 55

Angiotensin Converting Enzyme

(ACE) Inhibitors

Mechanism of Action

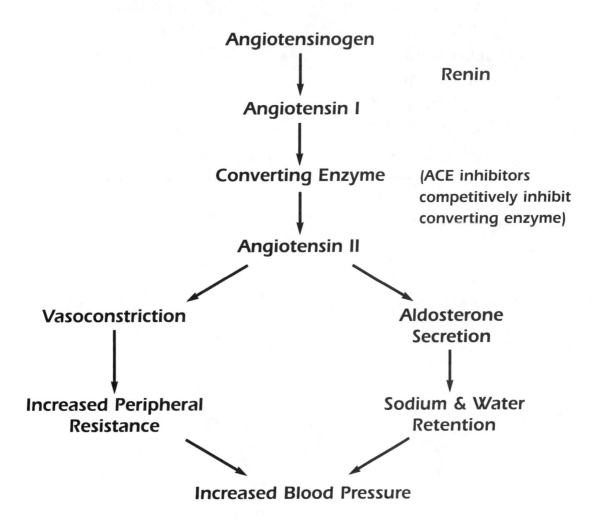

Angiotensinogen

Renin

Angiotensin I

Converting Enzyme   (ACE inhibitors competitively inhibit converting enzyme)

Angiotensin II

Vasoconstriction   Aldosterone Secretion

Increased Peripheral Resistance   Sodium & Water Retention

Increased Blood Pressure

Chapter 55

Angiotensin Converting Enzyme (ACE) Inhibitors

Generic Name	Trade Name
Benazepril	Lotensin
Captopril	Capoten
Enalapril	Vasotec
Fosinopril	Monopril
Lisinopril	Prinivil, Zestril
Moexipril	Univase
Quinapril	Accupril
Ramipril	Altace
Trandolapril	Mavik

Chapter 55

Comparison of Heparin and Warfarin (Coumadin)

	Heparin	Coumadin
Indications for Use	Acute thromboembolic problems Prophylaxis for clients at risk	Long-term treatment or prevention
Onset	Rapid, within minutes	Delayed 2 to 5 days
Duration	Short	2 to 5 days after discontinued
Route	IV, SC	PO
Blood Tests	Activated partial thromboplastin time (APTT)	Prothrombin time (PT) International Normalized Ratio (INR)
Antidote	Protamine sulfate	Vitamin K

Chapter 57

Anti-Ulcer Drugs

Antacids

Maalox, Mylanta, others

Antibacterials

Amoxicillin (Amoxil)
Clarithromycin (Biaxin)
Metronidazole (Flagyl)
Tetracycline (Sumycin)

Histamine$_2$ Receptor Antagonists

Cimetidine (Tagamet)
Famotidine (Pepcid)
Nizatidine (Axid)
Ranitidine (Zantac)

Prostaglandin

Misoprostol (Cytotec)

Proton Pump Inhibitors

Lansoprazole (Prevacid)
Omeprazole (Prilosec)

Miscellaneous

Bismuth subsalicylate (Pepto-Bismol)
Sucralfate (Carafate)

Chapter 60

Types of Anticancer Drugs

Alkylating Agents

Antimetabolites

Antibiotics

Plant Alkaloids

Hormones

Antihormones

Miscellaneous